THE 50+ WELLNESS

PROGRAM

THE 50+ WELLNESS PROGRAM

Harris H. McIlwain, M.D.
Lori F. Steinmeyer, M.S., R.D.
Debra Fulghum Bruce
R. E. Fulghum, Health Administrator
Robert G. Bruce, Jr., M.Div.

WILEY

John Wiley & Sons, Inc.
New York • Chichester • Brisbane • Toronto • Singapore

Library of Congress Cataloging-in-Publication Data

The 50+ wellness program / Harris H. McIlwain ... [et. a lp2.
     p.   cm.
   Includes bibliographical references.
   ISBN 0-471-50686-9 (pbk.)
   1. Aged—Health and hygiene. 2. Middle aged—Health and hygiene.
I. McIlwain, Harris H. II. Title: The 50 plus wellness program.
RA564.8.A15 1989
613'.0438—dc20   89-16563
                                      CIP

Printed in the United States of America

90 91 10 9 8 7 6 5 4 3 2 1

To those who wish
to live all their years to the fullest,
and in the spirit of thanks to Jewel Holden Fulghum
and Eddie and Cordelia McIlwain

Acknowledgments

We would especially like to thank the following health care professionals for their outstanding knowledge, personal contributions, and continued interest in *The 50+ Wellness Program*. Without the following people, this book would never have been possible:

Rand W. Altemose, M.D.
St. Joseph's Hospital
Tampa, Florida

Michael C. Burnette, M.D.
St. Joseph's Hospital
University Community Hospital
Tampa, Florida

Richard S. Eatroff, M.D.
Humana Hospital Brandon
Brandon, Florida

Will G. Harris, M.D., F.A.C.O.G.
St. Joseph's Hospital
Humana Women's Hospital
Tampa, Florida

James A. Holliday, Jr., M.D.
Assistant Clinical Professor
Department of Surgery
Section of Otolaryngology
College of Medicine
University of South Florida
St. Joseph's Hospital
Tampa, Florida

James E. McIlwain, Jr., D.D.S.,
  M.S.D.
Clinical Associate Professor
School of Dentistry
University of Florida
St. Joseph's Hospital
Tampa, Florida

Al Mooney, M.D.
Director
Willingway Hospital
Statesboro, Georgia

Joseph P. Nicoletto, M.D.
Chief of Urology and Surgical
  Subspecialties
University Community Hospital
Tampa, Florida

Thomas J. Pusateri, M.D.
Clinical Associate Professor
Department of Opthamology
College of Medicine
University of South Florida
University Community Hospital
Tampa, Florida

Joel C. Silverfield, M.D.
St. Joseph's Hospital
University Community Hospital
Tampa, Florida

Mac Steinmeyer, M.Div.
United Methodist Church
Tallahassee, Florida

Gerald L. Stoker, M.D.
Clinical Associate Professor
  of Medicine
Section of Dermatology
College of Medicine
University of South Florida
St. Joseph's Hospital
Tampa, Florida

James A. Wessman, C.P.A.
Partner - Thomas Craig &
  Company
Certified Public Accountants
Tampa, Florida

Angus Williams, Senior Agent
Principal Mutual Life Insurance
  Company
Tampa, Florida

Trademarks

Achromycin is a trademark of Lederle Laboratories, Division of American Cyanamide Company

Adapin is a trademark of Pennwalt Prescription Division, Pennwalt Corporation

Adriamycin is a trademark of Adria Laboratories, Division of Erbamont, Inc.

Advil is a trademark of Whitehall Laboratories, Inc., Division of American Home Products Corporation

Aldactone is a trademark of Searle and Company

Alka-Seltzer is a trademark of Miles Laboratories, Inc.

Amphojel is a trademark of Wyeth Laboratories, Division of American Home Products Corporation

Apresoline Hydrochloride is a trademark of CIBA Pharmaceutical Company, Division of CIBA-GEIGY Corporation

Bactrim DS is a trademark of Roche Laboratories, Division of Hoffmann-La Roche, Inc.

Benadryl is a trademark of Parke-Davis, Division of Warner-Lambert Company

Bicillin is a trademark of Wyeth Laboratories, Division of American Home Products Corporation

Blenoxane is a trademark of Bristol-Myers Oncology Division, Bristol-Myers Company

Bran Chex is a trademark of Ralston Purina Company

Capoten is a trademark of E. R. Squibb and Sons, Inc.

Cardizem is a trademark of Marion Laboratories, Inc.

Carnation Instant Breakfast is a trademark of the Carnation Company

Catapres is a trademark of Boehringer Ingelheim Pharmaceuticals, Inc., a subsidiary of Boehringer Ingelheim Corporation

Ceclor is a trademark of Eli Lilly and Company

Chlor-trimeton is a trademark of Schering Corporation

Colace is a trademark of Mead Johnson Pharmaceutical Division, Mead Johnson and Company

Cosmegen injection is a trademark of Merck, Sharp and Dohme, Division of Merck and Company, Inc.

Cracklin Bran is a trademark of the Kellogg Company
Crispex is a trademark of the Kellogg Company
Coumadin is a trademark of Du Pont Pharmaceuticals
Cuprimine is a trademark of Merck, Sharp and Dohme, Division of Merck and Company, Inc.
Cytoxan is a trademark of Bristol-Myers Oncology Division, Bristol-Myers Company
Datril is a trademark of Bristol-Myers Products, Division of Bristol-Myers Company
Dilantin is a trademark of Parke-Davis, Division of Warner-Lambert Company
Doxinate is a trademark of Hoechst-Roussel Pharmaceuticals, Inc.
Elavil is a trademark of Merck, Sharp and Dohme, Division of Merck and Company, Inc.
E-Mycin is a trademark of The Upjohn Company
Enrich is a trademark of Ross Laboratories, Division of Abbott Laboratories
Ensure is a trademark of Ross Laboratories, Division of Abbott Laboratories
Ensure Plus is a trademark of Ross Laboratories, Division of Abbott Laboratories
Erythrocin stearate is a trademark of Abbott Pharmaceuticals, Inc.
Feen-A-Mint is a trademark of Plough, Inc.
Fluorouracil is a trademark of Roche Laboratories, Division of Hoffman-La Roche, Inc.
40% Bran Flakes is a trademark of Publix Supermarkets, Inc.
Frosted Mini Wheats is a trademark of the Kellogg Company
Fruit Loops is a trademark of the Kellogg Company
Golden Grahams is a trademark of General Mills, Inc.
Honey Smacks is a trademark of the Kellogg Company
Hydrodiuril is a trademark of Merck Sharp and Dohme, Division of Merck and Company, Inc.
Inderal is a trademark of Ayerst Laboratories, Division of American Home Products
    Corporation
Indocin is a trademark of Merck, Sharp and Dohme, Division of Merck and Company, Inc.
Isoptin is a trademark of Knoll Pharmaceutical Company
Keflex is a trademark of Dista Products Company, Division of Eli Lilly and Company
Klor is a trademark of Upsher Smith Laboratories, Inc.
K-lyte is a trademark of Mead Johnson Laboratories, Mead Johnson Company
Lanoxin is a trademark of Burroughs Wellcome Company
Lasix is a trademark of Hoechst-Roussel Pharmaceuticals, Inc.
Levo thyroxine Sodium is a trademark of Lederle Laboratories, Division of American
    Cyanamid Company
Luminal is a trademark of Winthrop-Breon Laboratories
Meretene is a trademark of Sandoz, Inc.
Morton Lite Salt is a trademark of Morton Salt Division, of Morton Thiokol, Inc.
Maalox is a trademark of William H. Rorer, Inc.
Marplan is a trademark of Roche Laboratories, Division of Hoffman-La Roche, Inc.
Methotrexate is a trademark of Lederle Laboratories, Division of American Cyanamid
    Company
Minipress is a trademark of Pfizer Laboratories, Division of Pfizer, Inc.
Motrin is a trademark of The Upjohn Company
Mustagen is a trademark of Merck, Sharp and Dohme, Division of Merck and Company, Inc.
Naprosyn is a trademark of Syntex Laboratories, Inc.
Nardil is a trademark of Parke-Davis, Division of Warner-Lambert Company
Nitro-bid is a trademark of Marion Laboratories, Inc.
Nitroglyn is a trademark of Key Pharmaceuticals, Inc.
Nuprin is a trademark of Bristol-Myers Products, Division of Bristol-Myers Company
Nutrific Oatmeal is a trademark of the Kellogg Company
Oncovin is a trademark of Eli Lilly and Company
Oretic is a trademark of Abbott Pharmaceuticals, Inc.
Orinase is a trademark of the Upjohn Company
Parnate is a trademark of Smith, Kline and French Laboratories, Division of SmithKline
    Beckman Corporation

Pepto-Bismol is a trademark of Proctor and Gamble

Periactin is a trademark of Merck, Sharp and Dohme, Division of Merck and Company, Inc.

Persantine is a trademark of Boehringer Ingelheim Pharmaceuticals, Inc., a subsidiary of Boehringer Ingelheim Corporation

Penicillin G Potassium (oral) is a trademark of Lederle Laboratories, Division of American Cyanide Company

Phentoin Sodium is a trademark of Schein Pharmaceuticals, Inc.

Polycillin is a trademark of Bristol Laboratories, Division of Bristol-Myers Company

Premarin is a trademark of Ayerst Laboratories, Division of American Home Products Corporation

Procardia is a trademark of Pfizer Laboratories, Pfizer, Inc.

Questran is a trademark of Mead Johnson Pharmaceuticals, Mead Johnson and Company

Resource is a trademark of Sandoz, Inc.

Rice Krispies is a trademark of the Kellogg Company

Rolaids is a trademark of Warner-Lambert Company

Septra is a trademark of Burroughs Wellcome Company

Sinequan is a trademark of Roerig, Division of Pfizer Pharmaceuticals

Sugar Frosted Flakes is a trademark of the Kellogg Company

Surfak is a trademark of Hoechst-Roussel Pharmaceuticals, Inc.

Sustacal is a trademark of Mead Johnson Nutritional Division, Mead Johnson and Company

Sustacal High Calorie is a trademark of Mead Johnson Nutritional Division, Mead Johnson and Company

Sustagen is a trademark of Mead Johnson Nutrition Division, Mead Johnson and Company

Tagamet is a trademark of Smith Kline and French Laboratories, Division of SmithKline Beckman Corporation

Tolinase is a trademark of the Upjohn Company

Total is a trademark of General Mills, Inc.

Tums is a trademark of Norcliff Thayer, Inc.

Tylenol is a trademark of McNeil Consumer Products

Velban is a trademark of Eli Lilly and Company

Zyloprim is a trademark of Burroughs Wellcome Company

Contents

• Anemia • Anxiety • Arthritis • Asthma • Back Pain
• Bell's Palsy • Bronchitis (Acute) • Bronchitis (Chronic)
• Bursitis • Cancer • Carpal Tunnel Syndrome • Cataracts
• Chest Pain or Chest Discomfort • Coronary Heart
Disease • Cold (Rhinitis) • Cough • Dementia • Dental
Care • Depression • Diabetes Mellitus • Dizziness • Drug
Abuse • Dry Eyes • Dryness of the Mouth • Ear Noise
(Tinnitus) • Epistaxis (Nosebleed) • Eye Disorders • Facial
Wrinkles • Facial Pain • Fainting (Syncope) • Fatigue
• Fever • Fibrositis • Floaters • Glaucoma • Gout • Gum
Disease • Gynecological Concerns • Hair Loss • Headache
• Hearing Loss • Heart Failure • Hoarseness • Hypoglycemia
• Incontinence and Bladder Control • Insomnia—Difficulty
Sleeping and Daytime Sleepiness • Jaw Pain • Joint Pains
• Kidney Stones • Leg Pain • Lumps in the Neck • Macular
Degeneration • Mouth • Obesity (Overweight) • Osteoarthritis
• Osteoporosis • Palpitations • Pneumonia • Polymyalgia
Rheumatica • Prostate Diseases • Rheumatoid Arthritis
• Rhinitis—Caused by Medication • Sexual Problems (Sexual
Dysfunction) • Shortness of Breath • Skin Changes • Skin
Cancer • Skin Moles (Nevi) • Skin Infections • Snoring
• Sore Throat (Pharyngitis) • Stroke (Cerebrovascular
Accident) • Swallowing Difficulty (Dysphagia) • Systemic
Lupus Erythematosus • Swelling (Edema) • Temporal
Arteritis • Tendonitis • Thyroid Disease • Blood in
Urine (Hematuria) • Urinary Tract Infection • Weight
Loss • Wheezing •

INTRODUCTION
The Mature Years Are the Best Years

The mature years can be the best years. You are more experienced and knowledgeable than at any other point in your life. These years are to be celebrated as you make the choices you want in activities, involvement, different careers, residence, and more. Only by understanding the changes that are taking place internally and externally during the mature years can you feel free to make these choices.

The 50+ Wellness Program is not meant to be a medical encyclopedia and in no way can it replace good medical care by your physician, but it will give you a wealth of information. If you know the facts, you can begin to take charge of your health and your life.

Research shows that people who take control of their bodies and lifestyle are healthier and make fewer demands for high-cost hospitalization. As you study the information given in this health care guide, you will be able to control many of the problems that are likely to develop as you mature.

Remember, maturity is not a disease! Maturing is a natural process that happens to everyone, but you can take charge of certain aspects of aging by reducing risk factors for diseases, detecting certain problems early, maintaining a healthful diet, keeping physically and mentally active, and thinking positively. By extending good health past middle age, you can have the highest expectations for fulfilling mature years.

The goal of this book is to help you understand the facts of becoming a mature adult. It will help you recognize which changes you can prevent, which changes must happen whether you like them or not, and which changes can be ignored. This information can help take much of the uncertainty and fear away from the idea of becoming a mature adult. You will be able to see some of the problems of maturity that can be prevented long before they become apparent.

There is no magic way to know what action should be taken to prevent certain problems. When you know the facts, you can take charge to begin to manage your maturity with a plan so you can remain healthier, more active, and more in control of the future. You will be able to take advantage of those abilities that improve as we grow older, making your life more effective and gratifying.

The 50+ Wellness Program offers you a *holistic* approach to growing older. The book discusses all aspects of aging including health problems, physical symptoms, nutritional needs, financial planning, and life changes in the mature years. We feel that all of these factors combine to determine the overall health and well-being of the mature adult. If you are in control of all aspects of your life, it is much more likely that your quality of living will be greatly enhanced.

This book emphasizes three key points in gaining control over your lifestyle as you mature:

1. Eliminating risk factors
2. Formulating a plan for healthy living
3. Responding to life changes

Throughout this guide, we have listed those *risk factors* that add to a person's chances of having a specific health problem. These risk factors need to be evaluated and special efforts made to eliminate those over which you have control. We have also stressed the importance of developing a plan in your life. This could involve a personal fitness plan, a nutritional plan, an individual medical exam plan, a retirement financial plan, a crisis plan for illness and death, a plan for positive living, and more. Taking charge of one's lifestyle involves *planning*. Once you have eliminated risk factors, then plans must be made to maintain your good health so your mature years will be quality years.

We have offered you a hands-on approach to understanding the many needs of aging. Using a variety of checklists, questionnaires, diagrams, and more, you can use this guide as a learning tool as well as a place to keep your personal medical records. We urge you to fill in the questionnaires, use the checklists to evaluate your life, take the quizzes, then use this information to improve your quality of living as you develop your personal plan for good health.

■ UNDERSTANDING BALANCED NUTRITION

This book will give you insight into the benefits of good nutrition and how it effects the health and energy level of the mature adult.

Disease prevention and management depend on balanced nutrition in the daily diet. Once you understand the nutrient values of the foods you need each day, you can plan healthful menus with your longevity in mind.

■ UNDERSTANDING FINANCIAL SECURITY

Because added stress and worry can greatly effect one's emotional and physical health, this book will give you information on how to establish financial security during the mature adult years using your present resources, your retirement fund, and available government services. Medicare, Medicaid, Social Security, and other vital sources will be explained in detail as you make a comprehensive plan of your financial status for retirement.

■ PREVENTION: ELIMINATING RISK FACTORS

Throughout this book, we will emphasize the importance of starting today with preventive measures that could determine the quality of your life during retirement years.

We recently saw a 53-year-old woman in our clinic who was concerned because her mother had died a few months after she suffered a broken hip due to osteoporosis. Osteoporosis is a condition in which bones become thinner and are much more likely to break. This 53-year-old woman had learned that certain risk factors make a person much more likely than others to develop osteoporosis. She found that by removing some of these risk factors, by stopping smoking, adding estrogen treatment after menopause, and starting a weight-bearing exercise program, she would greatly reduce her risk of osteoporosis and hip fractures in future years. While still in her mid-life years, she is wisely preparing for mature adulthood by making changes in her lifestyle that will benefit her health and activity level in later years.

The 50+ Wellness Program will tell you what to expect—the signs and the feelings of becoming a mature adult. We will help you try to tell normal events from signs of more serious problems. You will learn which changes should not be accepted, including physical and emotional changes, and how to control them.

Prevention is definitely available for many of the problems encountered in maturity. The most common cause of death in the United States is heart disease, specifically coronary heart disease in which blockage develops in the blood vessels that supply blood to the heart itself. Certain risk factors are known to make a person much more likely to have heart disease. The more risk factors you have, the greater your chances of having coronary heart disease. The good news is that if you do have these risk factors and remove them, you lower your risk of developing coronary heart disease. You can actually change your future health by knowing what to do many years earlier.

Other diseases can also be prevented or decreased in severity if certain actions are taken. These will be discussed in later chapters.

What about the routine medical exam? When should you start having regular checkups? Or is it necessary to do this at all? It turns out that certain examinations are very easy and greatly help in early detection and treatment of problems (such as cancer) which can be very serious if ignored.

Suggestions to help answer these questions, to help know when to ask your physician questions, and when to think about a second opinion are also covered in *The 50+ Wellness Program*.

Some of the most common medical problems in the mature adult including signs and feelings, tests commonly ordered, and possible treatments are discussed. These problems include heart disease, stroke, arthritis, and others. Suggestions are made for actions you should take when you notice certain problems such as headache, dizziness, fever, chest pain, rashes, weight loss, memory changes, and other problems. Some specific problems are very important with action needed as early as possible. Others are less important and might wait until your next contact with your physician.

■ KNOWING THE FACTS ABOUT MATURE ADULTS

The proportion of our population in their mature years is larger than ever before. In 1900, there were 3 million people age 65 and older in the United States (about 4 percent of the entire U.S. population). In 1988, this figure increased to approximately 39.7 million Americans. By the year 2020, the Census Bureau projects that there will be 70 million Americans aged 55 and older (20 percent of Americans).

Are there any of us who are not bothered a little when we think of growing older? What about when we reach one of the landmark birthdays of 30, 40, 50, or 60? If we thought 30 seemed old, remember the black balloons friends sent for the "Over-the-Hill" party at 40?

Let's face it. For most of us, thoughts of leaving our youth and growing older create anxiety and fears. Some adults worry about the things that can happen with age, such as changes in looks, serious illnesses, loss of abilities, loneliness, and death. Many adults begin to confuse some of the normal changes in their bodies with changes caused by diseases. Some may think that it is necessary to become less useful and active as they grow older. Worries about eating the right foods to prevent diseases or about changes in diet requirements begin to add to these other health anxieties. Financial worries may top the list as some people dread retirement and having to live on a limited income.

You can take comfort in knowing that these are all common fears. The good news is that many of these fears can be greatly eased when you learn the facts. Many of the changes we see in our bodies are, in fact, the result of maturity. Most of these signs are normal events that in no way predict any future disease, loss of ability, or death. You may remember some of these signs of aging in an older friend or relative who died, even though there was no true connection between the signs of maturity and the cause of death. Lack of knowledge of the facts of aging may cause much unnecessary stress and worry.

For example, a 55-year-old woman was worried because she noticed some areas of bruising over the back of her hands. She knew that her mother had bruises over her arms and legs before she died of leukemia and was concerned that this was a sign of a serious blood disease. She was not aware that it is very common for normal persons to have small areas of bruised-appearing skin over the hands. This is thought to be caused by changes in tissue with more fragile blood vessels as we grow older. Some people show this change more than others, but it is not at all related to a serious blood disease or leukemia.

Another patient was extremely worried about a cough she had noticed over a few weeks. She had no serious illness and the cough quickly disappeared with treatment. But her main fear and the reason she saw a physician was because she knew that her mother had a cough when she died of heart failure. It is true that a cough can happen in heart failure, but it is only one of many, much more important signs that true heart disease is present.

Some changes may lead to serious illness if ignored. Becoming overweight, having high blood pressure, and ignoring certain changes in skin moles may each cause serious problems later when they are much less treatable.

■ UNDERSTANDING THE CHANGES OF MATURING

Because of the vast improvement in health care over the past 90 years including more prevention and treatment of diseases, our life span has increased greatly. Because we are living longer lives, many people are concerned about the quality of these extra years. Most of us do not look forward to spending added years of our lives as unhappy, sick, or lonely older adults. Most of us do not want to be a burden to our families or society because of prolonged illness or inadequate financial planning. Simply adding years to a person's life is not acceptable to people approaching retirement years. The goal should be to make those extra years as enjoyable, fulfilling, and productive as possible.

In many cases, we can have enough control of our own health to make a major difference in later years. For example, prevention of heart attacks and strokes, prevention of bone fractures, and early detection and treatment of cancer are all reasonable goals. It is true that some diseases cannot be prevented, but it is also true that the most common causes of serious illness and death in America today have good possibilities for prevention and early detection. You must know what to do to allow this prevention and early treatment.

If we could control those diseases that limit us in the later years, we would be able to live those years with much more enjoyment and personal fulfillment. We would also remain productive in our mature years. More of our lives would be spent in the ways we choose—not dependent, unhappy, or lonely.

Yes, many mature adults require more medical care and treatment than young adults. This means that our nation's health care bill will likely increase significantly over the next 20 years. If we could prevent illness and detect treatable illnesses early, then we would probably greatly decrease our health care costs.

If you know what to do, which steps to follow in prevention and early detection of health problems, you can begin to have more control over your future health. You will be able to feel comfortable that you are doing all that you can to prevent future problems.

☐ *PART I*

Eliminating Risk Factors

CHAPTER 1

Signs and Symptoms of Aging

The state of your health may be closely associated with your lifestyle. The federal government's Office of Disease Prevention and Health Promotion estimates that an unhealthy lifestyle accounts for 50 percent of the deaths before age 65. Because increased longevity and quality of life is important to you, responsibility must be taken by you to make the necessary lifestyle adjustments. You can begin to manage your lifestyle with a step-by-step evaluation of your current health status. Heredity and living environment are risk factors that need to be taken seriously as well as making new goals with your body's particular needs in mind. These goals might involve changes in activity, diet, and overall daily habits.

As you make this in-depth study of your current health, one challenge is to separate the body's normal changes which are not dangerous from new problems that are true signs of underlying disease. There are very specific changes as you grow older. Some change the way you look, but do not change the way you function or work. Let's look at some of the common signs and symptoms of the aging process.

■ SIGNS AND SYMPTOMS

No one escapes the changes that come with age. Some changes are welcome events such as improvement in a work situation and position, improved financial condition, new personal and social contacts. Yet some changes are less welcome, especially the changes that remind us that our bodies are aging. Once we allow ourselves to accept that these changes cannot be avoided, we can begin to manage these changes so that they do not limit us. Many of the changes, such as the graying of hair or facial wrinkles, do not create problems. Rather it is what these changes mean to us that causes anxiety. We take these changes to be signs of old age, and in our minds old age means less activity, poor health, and death.

Many of these changes in appearance are in fact signs of becoming a mature adult, but most changes *do not* mean that infirmity will soon follow. It is very important that we learn to tell which changes are incidental, which are unavoidable, and which can be ignored. For example, facial wrinkles are common and usually increase with age and maturity. In some persons, wrinkles occur earlier in life for no explainable reason. In others, wrinkles may occur because of more sun exposure in earlier years. Wrinkles alone do not have any connection with other diseases. They are simply part of the maturing process.

Remember that changes in one part of the body as we mature (such as facial wrinkles) do not predict changes in other parts of the body, such as the heart or brain. Usually each system of organs has its own rate of change. We cannot generalize and assume that because there is a problem in one area that other organs will be affected also. The rate of changes taking place during the maturing process may vary greatly among the organs in the same person. For example, the skin may show many signs of aging while the heart and lungs remain nearly normal.

■ PEOPLE MATURE AT DIFFERENT RATES

One way to understand how the changes that accompany maturity vary among people is to think about the changes of growth and maturity in children. One child may show changes of growth and maturity earlier than others. The rate of development varies even in the same child at different times. For example, one child develops a first tooth at 3 months, another at 12 months, or one child reaches puberty at 12 years, another at 14 years. In the same way, adults mature at different rates. Some systems in an adult may not show signs of aging and maturity as rapidly as others. Chronological age alone does not predict which changes of maturity have happened; it certainly *does not* predict abilities accurately. Remember that Colonel Sanders began a successful chicken restaurant after age 65, and Arthur Rubenstein was still a concert pianist at age 90!

Each change that comes with maturity can be managed separately. Some changes may indicate a potential problem, but not all changes are red flags. If you can identify the changes that indicate problems, you can take action early to avoid some of the problems. How do you tell the difference? There are reasonable ways to help decide what action to take. Later chapters in this book explain which changes to notice and what to do when you find new problems.

■ NOTICEABLE SIGNS OF AGING

Skin changes are some of the first noticed changes of aging. This is also an area in which the effects of outside forces on maturity are easily seen. Among the normal changes to the skin are changes in the number of pigment cells. The number of these cells (called melanocytes) decreases gradually after about age 30. Since these are the pigment-containing cells, there is eventually a decrease in the ability to tan as evenly as before. The groups of remaining pigment cells may look more prominent—they appear as spots over the arms or face and have been called "age spots." These are harmless changes in the skin color. They may become darker and more noticeable with more sun exposure.

Some layers of the skin become thinner with age, especially in women. Changes in the fibers that make up the skin also make the skin strength change in such a way that the skin tears more easily and bruises occur more readily. This is most often seen in areas of the body that receive normal everyday minor injuries—the back of the hands, the arms below the elbows, and the lower legs.

Changes in the fibers and thickness of the skin also mean that the skin becomes looser and wrinkles. Over the years, there is a decrease in the number of blood vessels in the superficial layers of the skin in the upper part of the body. This may give a paler appearance to the skin, especially in the face.

The number of sweat glands in the skin decreases with age. Also, the *sebaceous* glands make less secretions, contributing to the rough, dry skin that is common in older persons. The body becomes less efficient at keeping the skin moist and smooth.

Many of these normal changes in skin are brought on earlier or made more severe by large amounts of sun exposure. Wrinkling, dryness, changes in skin color, and easier bruising are commonly seen in persons who have had much sun exposure over the years. This is a good example of how an outside force can affect the rate of normal aging changes in the skin. Persons having much less sun exposure will still show these changes, but they may occur many years later or may be less drastic. Prolonged sun exposure also increases the risk of certain skin cancers (see the discussion on p. 220).

The rate of growth of fingernails and toenails begins to slow after age 25 to 30. The nails may eventually become thinner, softer, and more brittle. Ridges may develop along the length of the nail at the base. In older persons, the toenails may become thickened from age or disease. Calluses and changes in the bones of the foot may result in more foot discomfort.

Height

The belief that older people become shorter is true. Many researchers have measured the height of adults over a period of years. Some have estimated an average loss of about 1.2 cm (less than 0.5 in.) every 20 years after reaching maturity. The loss of height is mainly due to loss of height of the vertebral bodies in the spine (Fig. 1). These bones become shorter due to osteoporosis and can appear compressed on an x-ray of the spine, causing the spine to become shorter and stooped (Fig. 2). Another cause of loss of height is narrowing of the disc between the

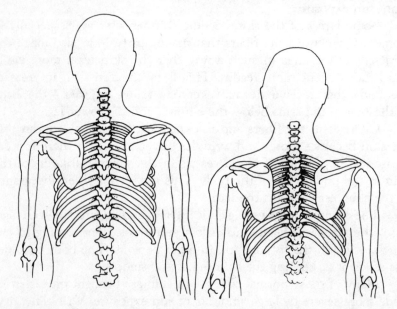

FIGURE 1   Loss of height due to spinal shortening.

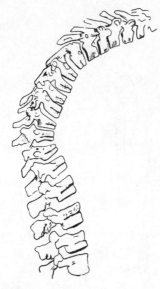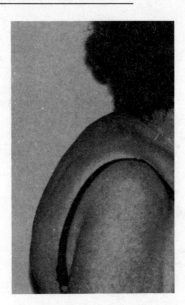

FIGURE 2 Dowager's hump.

vertebral bodies. If a person's posture becomes stooped or if the knees are slightly bent then loss of height will be even greater (Fig. 3).

Weight

Weight generally increases as adults mature, with the average peaking at ages 40 to 60. The average weight levels out in ages 65 to 75 and then usually gradually declines (Fig. 4).

The weight loss later in life is in part due to the loss of muscle throughout the body. The total amount of muscle gradually decreases with age. Accompanying this loss is a loss in strength as measured by handgrip strength. This is true for both men and women. These changes alone are not a sign of underlying disease.

Changes in the Face

Wrinkles are one of the earliest signs of maturity and aging in the face, generally starting with the forehead. Other common areas are wrinkles radiating from the corners of the eyes and wrinkles around the lips. If there is a loss of teeth, wrinkles around the mouth and lips may become more prominent.

Because the skin becomes looser over the face, there may be sagging of the skin of the eyelids, especially the upper eyelids. The

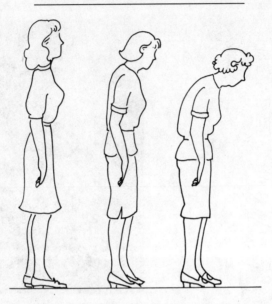

FIGURE 3 Comparison sketch of a young woman, middle-age woman, and elderly woman showing bending of spine due to osteoporosis with loss of height.

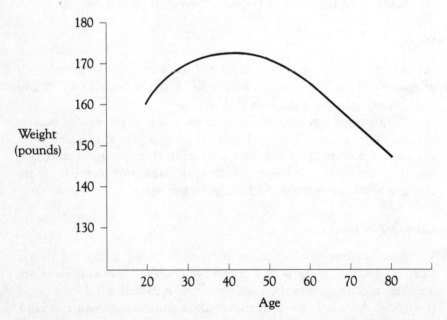

FIGURE 4 Some researchers have found that body weight often peaks around age 40–45, then may gradually decrease with age.

skin under the chin and the front of the neck may also become looser and draped in appearance.

The fat tissue under the skin over the face decreases with age, resulting in more prominent facial features with more prominent bones. The eyes may appear more sunken because of the loss of fat tissue around the eyes. These are normal changes that happen to some degree in all of us. The time of onset of these changes and the degree of change are what varies.

The same changes that result in looseness of the skin over the face also affect the skin of the ear. The cartilage structure of the ear changes very little, but the skin forming the ear lobe becomes looser and the ear increases in size. One researcher found that by age 80 many ears had increased in length by as much as 1.2 cm (less than 0.5 in.).

The blood vessels in the skin of the face, as well as other areas of the body, decrease in number as we mature. This may give the appearance of a paler face.

Abdomen Size

The size of the abdomen often gradually increases after ages 35 to 45. This is in part due to more fat deposits in the abdomen fat storage sites, even though the total weight of the body may decline. Less physical activity with weaker abdominal muscles, stooped posture in some persons with osteoporosis in the spine, and other factors also can contribute to a larger abdominal measurement. This is not a sign of other diseases. It is a common part of aging. Measures to minimize these changes include a regular exercise program discussed on page 33.

Fat Tissue

Maturity brings loss of some of the fat tissue under the skin (called the subcutaneous fat). This is a gradual loss over many years. It may begin after ages 40 to 50. As a result, the bony prominences of the body—the spine, shoulder blades, facial bones, bones of the chest, and other bony structures may become more apparent. Loss of the fat tissue in a woman's breasts may change their appearance and make underlying glandular tissue more prominent. This may raise suspicion of abnormal growths and cancer. Even though these are quite normal happenings, the results can bring suspicions of some other disease or illness.

Hair

Graying of the hair over the body is common. It is caused by a decrease in the pigment cells which give the hair its color. The graying is usually gradual and may begin early in the 20s. Inherited factors play a role so that it is common to see several members of a family have early changes of hair color. Researchers estimate that about half of the population has graying of some hair over the body by age 50. More than half of the population over 50 has graying of the hair on the scalp.

Thinning of the hair is also common. The pattern of hair thinning in women is usually more generalized, with the top of the head often more severely involved. In men, the hair loss begins in the front part of the scalp and gradually extends to involve the crown and top of the scalp. Men usually don't lose hair along the fringe of the scalp. In fact, this is a source of hair for transplanting to other areas of the scalp.

Hair loss is common. It may be gradual over the scalp and throughout the body. This hair loss is often preceded by graying. Hair loss under the arms (axillary hair) also occurs normally in aging. The central hairs remain and are often grayer and thinner. Loss of axillary hair is common after about age 60. Pubic hair and hair on the legs and arms also may decrease in the aging process.

New hair may appear in some areas of the body. This hair is course, dark, and short. It may appear over the ears, nose, or eyebrows in men, with similar hair appearing over the chin in women. Some researchers have found that over 40 percent of all women in the age group of 75 to 84 have chin hair. These changes alone are not signs of other underlying diseases. They are normal changes of maturity.

Mouth and Teeth

The great concern of our childhood over cavity prevention to prevent tooth loss shifts to a great concern over the prevention of gum disease. Gum disease (periodontal disease) is the most significant cause of tooth loss in the mature adult. In this disease, the tissue that supports the teeth breaks down. This leads to tooth loss even though the tooth itself may be normal. Cavities become more common at the roots of the teeth instead of over the crown (Fig. 5). With tooth loss comes a change in the shape of the jaw.

The tooth enamel often becomes darker, a bit more yellow, and less translucent as we age. Compare the outer enamel layer of the tooth with porcelain. As porcelain ages, it develops thin lines which do not weaken the surface, but stains can occur in these lines. Stains

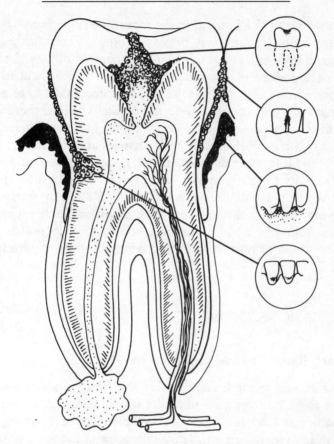

FIGURE 5 Adults often have secondary decay around old fillings and decay of tooth roots, which become exposed when the gums recede with age or due to periodontal disease.

will be more pronounced with heavy smoking or frequent drinking of coffee or tea.

As we get older, there is also a slight shifting of the tooth position. A space may occur between the teeth or tipping will gradually take place, particularly if any teeth are lost. Even after orthodontic treatment where the teeth are aligned in a nearly ideal position, changes occur over the years. A second correction could be considered in some instances.

There is a gradual recession of the gum tissues. The gum (gingival) tissue may recede as the supporting bone around the teeth recedes. The process can be speeded by lack of care or neglecting good dental health. This process is usually so gradual that the teeth should be useful as long as needed.

The skin over the lips and in the mouth becomes more fragile in the mature adult. Healing may be slower due to many factors. Dryness of the mouth is common due to less effective salivary glands.

These are some of the most important changes in *appearance* which commonly happen as we mature. It is important to remember that changes of aging in one area do not predict whether there will be changes in other areas; each of us seems to progress at a different rate. These changes are considered normal changes and do not usually by themselves indicate other diseases. In fact, none of these changes affect a person's ability to think, reason, or a person's creativity. Most of the changes are not preventable, but some may be slowed by certain practices. Review any new changes with your physician. Each person is an individual. Your physician is the best person to help decide which changes are those of normal aging and which changes require further evaluation.

■ INTERNAL SIGNS OF AGING

The Heart, Blood Vessels, and Exercise

The most recent research tells us that our cardiovascular system—our heart and blood vessels—normally should continue to work well as we mature as long as diseases do not interfere. It is wrong to assume that as we mature past age 50 our bodies cannot exercise well, including even vigorous exercise.

There are some small changes that can be measured in the way our heart and blood vessels perform as we mature. However, the overall amount of work and exercise that the heart can do decreases little in normal persons from aging alone. The maximum ability to exercise may be maintained to a significant degree in many cases even up to age 80! In older persons, some changes can be detected, such as the maximum heart rate (number of beats per minute). This heart rate does normally slow slightly in older people. However, the heart makes up for this in other ways so that the total amount of work possible may not be changed. In other words, if no other diseases are present, then the maximum amount of exercise or exercise capacity can be maintained as we mature.

This means that most of us are quite capable of exercise, even vigorous exercise, throughout the mature years. Problems other than aging alone may limit our activity and exercise. Inactivity and lack of regular exercise contribute to a further decrease in the ability to exercise. The longer a person continues to be inactive, the more trouble there will be when exercise is attempted. Old age may be blamed as the cause for limitation in exercise ability, but it may not be the culprit.

If no other diseases are present, mature adults should be able to maintain a reasonable exercise program. There is evidence that a regular exercise program may help *prevent* heart problems. In other words, maintaining a regular exercise program can help prevent the very heart problems that might cause limitation!

This does *not* mean that you should immediately begin a vigorous exercise program. This might not be safe, but it *does* mean that if no other diseases are present, a vigorous exercise program would be a reasonable goal. You should ask your physician what level of exercise is safe to begin (such as walking) and how fast you might try to increase the activity. Some persons can begin at more energetic levels than others. Some may require tests to be sure no other diseases are present that might make some exercises unsafe.

Most people can safely follow a regular exercise program if it is done in the correct way under supervision. This should include the proper level of exercise—not too much at first, then slowly increasing if tolerated. It is not important to begin at a high level; it is more important to be consistent and slowly increase the amount of exercise. If you notice any unusual tiredness, shortness of breath, heaviness, or discomfort in your chest, you should stop immediately and contact your physician.

"Circulation" Problems

Circulation problems in the legs may accompany maturity. However, there are many *different* problems that are commonly referred to as circulation problems. The most common affect the veins and the arteries in the legs.

Swelling of the feet and legs can be caused by decreased return of the blood and fluid from the feet and legs back toward the heart. In many cases, the blood supply to the feet from the arteries is normal, but the return of the blood and tissue fluid is slower so that swelling occurs in the feet or in the lower legs. This reduced flow can be caused by problems in the veins or in the lymph vessels that return the blood and fluid back to the heart from the feet and legs. The swelling is usually more noticeable after prolonged sitting such as on a long car ride or airline flight. This type of swelling usually disappears quickly as you become more active again.

You may be able to see small blue streaks, especially in the lower legs; these are veins. These veins may become larger or more prominent over a period of time. These changes alone are not dangerous and may indicate varicose veins. Simple measures such as avoiding prolonged sitting usually help prevent the swelling. If the swelling does not go away quickly or if there is pain or other limitation, you should contact your physician to see if a more serious problem is present.

Cramping, tightness, or other discomfort or pain in the legs, especially in the calf during walking or other activity is definitely not normal and should not be thought of as a normal part of maturity. Blockage of the arteries in the leg may cause this problem. It is a problem that should *not* be ignored. You should contact your physician. This problem is discussed further on page 204.

The Lungs

The lungs do show some changes with maturity, especially in older age groups. There are changes in the small air sacs and airways throughout the lungs making them less efficient. In fact, the actual level of oxygen in the blood normally slowly decreases with age in a predictable way. This happens in persons who have no other lung problems and who do not smoke. Of course, smoking and other problems may make these changes happen much more rapidly. Despite these measurable changes in the lungs, the overall performance of the lungs is usually maintained so that there should not be noticeable limitation by shortness of breath unless other problems happen. Changes of maturity and aging should not include shortness of breath at rest or with activity. If you notice such problems, you should contact your physician.

Stomach and Intestines

The esophagus, stomach, small intestine, and large intestine are part of the gastrointestinal system. Various feelings and symptoms from these areas are common in maturity and aging. Some changes might be interpreted as signs of disease when they are not; other changes are important and need medical evaluation.

The muscles of the esophagus (foodpipe to the stomach) may be affected by weakness with maturity and aging, but this rarely results in symptoms. If there is difficulty in swallowing, it should be discussed with your physician. Occasional "heartburn" may happen in otherwise normal persons due to acid from the stomach moving backward into the esophagus. This is due to relaxation of the valve separating the stomach and esophagus. If this happens frequently, it may indicate abnormal relaxation of the valve and require evaluation by your physician.

Many people develop indigestion, belching, and "gas." Abdominal pain and cramps, constipation, diarrhea, the need for frequent laxatives, hemorrhoids, blood in the stool, and dark stools are common problems. These symptoms may have no serious implications and may go away without treatment. The problem is that each of these may also be a sign of a much more serious disease. Peptic ulcer disease, diverticulitis, gall bladder disease, liver disease, and other serious problems may be present. Guessing the cause turns out to be wrong on many occasions. Delaying treatment may have serious consequences. If you have any new or persistent symptoms, you should contact your physician so that you can be reassured that no serious problem is present, or so that proper diagnosis and treatment can start.

The Brain

As we mature, there is a gradual loss of nerve cells from the brain and other areas of the body. Loss of nerve cells from the brain may begin as early as age 20 to 30 years and the size of the brain may also begin to decrease after age 30 to 40. This does *not* mean that our abilities change in any way. These are common physical changes in otherwise normal persons.

Some symptoms and problems may make us worry about more serious problems related to the health and function of the brain. For example, forgetfulness is common, but if the forgetfulness becomes a serious loss of memory and interferes with daily life, then it is not normal. The problem is that it is often difficult to decide at what point a harmless symptom becomes a more serious sign of underlying disease. Usually if the symptoms are brief, mild, and do not interfere with your daily life, then they are not a cause for alarm. If the same problem (such as forgetfulness) begins to limit your daily activities, then it may be a sign of more serious problems and you should see your physician. For example, occasionally misplacing your keys, forgetting your place in the parking lot, or forgetting a name are common in normal persons. But if forgetfulness extends to more important situations such as important decisions in your work, then it would interfere with daily living and could be a sign of a more serious cause of memory loss.

Some problems that are usually not important if they happen only occasionally are forgetting names of acquaintances or places during a busy schedule. Some problems that should cause more concern are forgetting the names of family members, frequently forgetting important dates, or directions to familiar places. If these happen, you should consider asking the advice of your physician to be sure there is not a more serious problem. Testing can help to tell the difference between "normal" forgetfulness and true signs of more serious problems (see p. 154).

Muscles and Joints

Aches and pains can occur at any age. Pain or stiffness without a known cause which lasts more than a few days is not a normal part of maturity or aging. If you have persistent pain or swelling in the joints, you should contact your physician. Other signs that are not explained by normal maturity or aging include stiffness in the muscles or joints in the morning that is severe or lasts several hours. Limitation of daily activities by pain in the muscles or joints or by weakness in the muscles is not a part of normal maturity or aging. Many of these problems could be caused by arthritis or related diseases. Often these sort of problems can be improved or prevented from becoming worse, especially if treatment is received early.

Eyes and Sight

We are all aware that our eyes change with age. Some changes are especially common in maturity and aging. These changes may begin as early as age 20. Some changes may be ignored, but some may interfere with daily activities. One common change is a decrease in the size of the pupil of the eye. As a result, less light is allowed into the eye. Some people may simply need a brighter source of light, but the condition becomes gradually more pronounced after age 30.

By the time one reaches 40, the eyes have increasing difficulty focusing up close. This is a normal aging change; the lens inside the eye is unable to focus on nearby objects. This condition is known as presbyopia and occurs with age to varying degrees in everyone. There is no exercise or medication that will reverse the process. "Reading" glasses or bifocals are often necessary although contact lenses may help. Everyone should have their vision checked at least every two years. If new glasses do not correct this problem, it is strongly recommended that a complete examination by an opthalmologist be done as soon as possible.

Many vision changes can be quite limiting for our daily activities even though they are normal in maturity. These problems are most commonly corrected with glasses or contact lenses. This is a good example of one part of aging that can be controlled. However, these changes in vision can also be caused by other more serious problems. It is very important to have a proper eye examination so that other eye problems can be detected early when treatment is most effective. A change in your vision should be reason to contact your ophthalmologist or optometrist.

Ears and Hearing

We all know an older person who has difficulty hearing. In fact, everyone usually suffers gradual decrease in their ability to hear sounds with increasing age. This may happen early or it may be delayed until advanced age. It is more common in men than in women. High tones are frequently more affected than low tones. Some people compensate for this hearing loss better than others, and the loss may go unnoticed.

Factors such as working in a noisy environment for many years may make hearing loss happen earlier. Another common problem is an increasing difficulty in distinguishing sounds; the person is able to hear but has difficulty understanding speech and other daily sounds. This problem is usually worse if there is a noisy environment.

Although these are common problems in maturity, there are other problems that appear similar but are caused by more serious diseases of the ear and other organs. A proper examination is necessary to be sure no other causes of hearing problems are present and to decide if a hearing aid will be effective. Many but not all cases of hearing loss and impairment can be helped by hearing aids. The best advice is to discuss it with your physician.

■ SUMMARY

Most of the changes in appearance that occur as we mature are normal and can be accepted. It is important to distinguish between changes that are inevitable and those which may not be normal. Once you begin to understand the natural maturing process, you can take steps to manage these changes so that they do not greatly affect your lifestyle.

CHAPTER 2

Prevention
and
Early Detection

Maintaining good health should be one of the most important goals as you mature. Success in every other area of your life may be very limited if you have poor health. Some diseases are much more common (and much more likely to affect you) than others. In fact, many of the diseases that are most likely to limit you have excellent prevention measures, and early detection is possible.

Prevention is a key word for the mature adult. Many problems may be avoided altogether by eliminating the specific risk factors. Prevention for many diseases should begin years before the actual problem appears. For example, prevention of atherosclerosis (hardening and narrowing) of the arteries, begins early in life—in childhood, teenage years, and young adult years. It is never too late, but prevention is most effective if begun early. Control of those risk factors which make a person more likely to develop atherosclerosis may prevent heart disease and strokes many years later.

Early detection of medical problems allows treatment when it is easier, more effective, and less expensive. For example, a simple, painless test can detect blood in the stool—and allows early treatment of cancer in the intestine long before it causes any other signs. Also, a mammogram (a breast x-ray) may allow detection of breast cancer before any other signs are present. This allows treatment before the cancer has a chance to spread.

Many people ask questions such as:

- How do I know what to do?
- What problems do I look for?
- How do I prevent or detect these problems?

It is not practical to actually test for all possible medical problems, but it is possible to focus our efforts on those certain medical problems that are *most likely to occur*. This can allow you to manage your future health in a reasonable way, with a minimum amount of time and in the most cost-effective way.

■ PREVENTION AND EARLY DETECTION

Three specific areas for prevention and early detection of common but serious medical problems are discussed in this chapter. This can greatly increase your control of the most common causes of serious illness and death in the United States. Most importantly, remember to identify risk factors:

1. Identify and control your risk factors for hardening and narrowing of the arteries (atherosclerosis). This will minimize your risk of heart disease, stroke, kidney failure, and other diseases.

2. Identify your risk factors for certain common types of cancer and follow simple early detection methods. There are ways to lower your risk of developing many of these kinds of cancer. For example, the risk of the most common kind of lung cancer can be largely eliminated if you do not smoke cigarettes. After smokers quit, their risk of lung cancer gradually decreases. There are ways to detect many of the common types of cancer early when treatment is effective. You can have reasonable control of cancer detection.

3. Especially in females, identify and remove your risk factors for osteoporosis. This disease affects 80 percent of women over age 65 and results in thinning of the bones. Because the bones are weaker, they fracture more easily, especially the hip, spine, and wrist. This is the most common cause of hip fracture in older women. Hip fractures in the United States cost over $7 billion each year.

Certain risk factors make a person much more likely to develop osteoporosis. These risk factors can be identified and removed to lower the risk (see page 55). Begin treatment early once osteoporosis is detected. This can lower your chance of future fractures, disability, and loss of your independence.

You can manage these three areas with the help of your physician. Control of the three areas need not require frequent visits to doctors or clinics and does not have to be expensive or time consuming. If problems are found then specific tests can be planned. This plan might not detect some uncommon or rare diseases, but there is often little prevention available for many of these problems anyway.

With an organized plan you can feel comfortable that you are doing the most possible for prevention and early detection for treatment of the medical problems that would be most likely to cause you serious illness or death. Let's briefly discuss each of these three areas and show how you can begin to manage your future health.

■ RISK FACTORS FOR ATHEROSCLEROSIS

Identify and review your risk factors for atherosclerosis. In atherosclerosis, the arteries become abnormally thickened and narrowed. If this process continues then the amount of blood that flows through the arteries is reduced. Eventually, the blood flow may be blocked completely. Since these arteries supply blood to the body's organs, they may not receive enough blood to allow them to work properly. The most common organs which are affected by this problem are the heart, brain, and kidney, resulting in heart attacks, heart failure, strokes, and kidney failure.

All of these problems can result in severe illness, limitation, and death. These diseases (especially coronary heart disease) are the most common cause of death in the United States. The process of hardening of the arteries builds up over many years. By the time a heart attack occurs, the disease has usually been present for years. In order to prevent this process, we must begin as early as possible.

Over the past 20 to 30 years, it has been found that atherosclerosis is not a necessary part of maturity and aging. Certain risk factors make a person much more likely to have atherosclerosis, especially in the coronary arteries where it can lead to heart attacks and heart failure. In the United States, over 500,000 people die due to coronary heart disease each year. The cost of cardiovascular disease is estimated to be over $78.6 billion each year!

You can lower your risk by reducing your risk factors. This can be done without spending a lot of time and money, but you must know specifically what to look for and how to change these risk factors. The risk factors for coronary heart disease which can be changed are:

1. High blood pressure (hypertension)
2. High blood cholesterol
3. Cigarette smoking
4. Regular exercise program
5. Excess body weight (obesity)
6. Stress management for hostility and anger
7. Control of diabetes mellitus

Risk factors which can't be changed are:

1. Family member with coronary heart disease before age 50
2. Age
3. Male sex

Let's review some of the most important risk factors and show how to remove or change them.

High Blood Pressure (Hypertension)

When the pressure measured in the arteries is abnormally high then the problem is called hypertension. It turns out that if a person has hypertension over a period of time (usually years), there is a much higher risk for other serious problems. The higher the blood pressure the higher the risk becomes. Insurance companies have known for years that elevated blood pressure will increase the risk of a person's future illness and early death.

It is known that the chance of hypertension increases with age. About ⅓ of adults in the United States have diastolic blood pressure above 85 or systolic blood pressure above 140. Up to ⅔ of persons ages 65 to 74 have elevated blood pressure.

If the blood pressure is lowered to normal levels, the risk of heart attack, stroke, heart failure, and kidney disease is also lowered. The earlier the treatment is begun, the more effective it will be in preventing disease. Detection of high blood pressure can be one of the most important steps to take in managing your health.

Over the past 20 years, there has been a 50 percent decrease in strokes and over 30 percent decrease in death from coronary heart disease. Control of hypertension is thought to be one important reason for these decreases. It is now estimated that over 50 million persons in the United States have hypertension. Control of the problem could greatly reduce the suffering and disability of other diseases, and would also greatly reduce our nation's health care bill. It is not difficult to detect and to treat hypertension. It can be done easily with a minimum of trouble and expense.

Many instruments are available to measure your blood pressure. The blood pressure is given in millimeters of mercury (mm Hg). In taking your blood pressure, two measurements are made. One is the *systolic* pressure (the upper number); the other is the *diastolic* pressure (the lower number). For example, a blood pressure of 120 mm Hg over 80 mm Hg is normal. Usually mm Hg is omitted and only the numbers are given such as "120 over 80" or written as 120/80.

There are a few points to remember when taking your blood pressure to make a more accurate reading. Read the instructions with your instrument if you are taking it at home. You should be sitting for a few minutes. Cigarettes, coffee, other caffeine products, and other medications that might raise blood pressure should be avoided if possible.

The size of the blood pressure cuff used on the arm is important. The standard size cuff fits most arms. If the cuff is too small for the arm size, the blood pressure may appear higher than it really is. If your arm is very large, you may need to use a larger size cuff (available at most medical supply stores). If you are not sure about the correct cuff to use, ask your physician for advice.

Many fire stations, shopping malls, pharmacies, and other stores now offer blood pressure measurements although some people like to have measurements taken at home. Three or 4 readings over a week or two weeks will give you a reasonable idea of your blood pressure. Record your blood pressure and the date it was taken so that you can tell if it changes later.

It is so easy to have blood pressure measured that we suggest checking the measurement 1 or 2 times each year if it remains normal. If it is elevated, it should be checked more often.

At what level is blood pressure too high? Systolic (upper number) blood pressure higher than 140 or diastolic (lower number) blood pressure higher than 90 are abnormal and raises the risk of future cardiovascular complications such as heart attack, stroke, heart failure, and kidney disease. The 1988 report of the Joint National Committee on Detection, Evaluation, and Treatment of High Blood Pressure offers guidelines for blood pressure readings in adults over 18 years old (Table 1).

TABLE 1
Blood Pressure Readings

Diastolic (Lower Number)

Less than 85 mm Hg	Normal blood pressure
85–89	High normal blood pressure
90–104	Mild hypertension
105–114	Moderate hypertension
115 or greater	Severe hypertension

Systolic (Upper Number) with Diastolic less than 90

Less than 140	Normal blood pressure
140–159	Borderline hypertension
160 or greater	Isolated systolic hypertension

One special problem of hypertension occurs in the mature adult. As the blood vessels mature (especially over age 60), they tend to become less elastic and flexible. They become more stiff and rigid. The blood pressure in the arteries may increase. Commonly in this situation, the systolic blood pressure increases more than the diastolic blood pressure. This is called *systolic hypertension.*

For many years it was thought that systolic hypertension was less important than diastolic hypertension. The "upper" number was thought to matter less than the "lower" number in blood pressure readings. It was thought that no treatment was needed in many cases. Now researchers have shown that systolic hypertension is at least as important as diastolic hypertension as a cause of future strokes, heart attacks, and other problems. Therefore, if the systolic blood pressure is consistently over 160 to 165, many physicians would favor treatment to lower the blood pressure to normal. The blood pressure can be controlled effectively and safely in most cases.

How might you feel if your blood pressure is high? Usually there are no symptoms at all. At some higher levels, headaches, dizziness, or signs of a stroke occur, but it is not safe to wait for these signs. In the majority of persons, no feelings are present to tell that your blood pressure is high.

If your blood pressure is above the normal range the Joint National Committee on Detection, Evaluation, and Treatment of High Blood Pressure have recommended the follow-up action listed in Table 2.

Choose the shorter time for follow up if your diastolic and systolic blood pressure give different recommended follow-up times

TABLE 2
Blood Pressure Readings and Follow-Up Recommendations

Diastolic Blood Pressure (Lower Number)	Recommended Follow-Up
Less than 85 mm Hg	Recheck within 2 years
85–89	Recheck within 1 year
90–104	See your physician
105–114	Needs evaluation within 2 weeks
Above 114	Needs evaluation immediately

(If Diastolic Blood Pressure less than 90)

Systolic Blood Pressure (Upper Number)	Recommended Follow-Up
Less than 140 mm Hg	Recheck within 2 years
140–199	See your physician
Over 199	Needs evaluation within 2 weeks

above. If your blood pressure is elevated but returns to normal after a few readings, it should be checked at least every 6 months.

These guidelines are the minimum needed for follow up of blood pressure. If you have other problems then you may need to have your blood pressure checked more often. Talk with your physician if your blood pressure is elevated or if you have any questions. The plan for evaluation and treatment can be made which best fits your own situation.

For example there are some uncommon medical problems that can cause hypertension but are often treatable. In fact, some medications can even cause hypertension. A few simple tests can show if any damage from the hypertension is present. Other risk factors for coronary heart disease may be present.

The goals of treatment are:

1. To reduce the blood pressure to normal range (or as close to normal as possible)
2. To control the blood pressure without side effects
3. If medications are used, to control blood pressure with the least expense possible and the fewest number of doses each day.

Many treatments are available for hypertension. These include treatment without medication and treatment using medication.

Suggestion: Measure your blood pressure at least yearly. If it is higher than 140 systolic (upper number) or higher than 90 diastolic (lower number), follow up is needed.

Treatment of Hypertension without Medication

Lower Your Salt Intake.   Many people who have hypertension can lower their blood pressure simply by lowering their sodium intake. It is not known why some persons are more sensitive to salt intake than others. Lowering the salt intake may allow you to avoid or take less medications. Since it is not very hard to reduce excess salt in the diet and since there are no serious side effects, this is an important part of controlling your blood pressure.

A few steps make it quite easy to reduce your sodium intake. First, don't add any salt to your food at the table. The food may still be cooked with a normal amount of salt—but don't cheat by increasing salt in cooking! Your taste will change so that you actually enjoy less salt. Soon the foods you used to enjoy will taste salty. This is a painless way to lower salt intake greatly for many of us. The more trouble you have breaking this salt habit, the more salt you may be taking in your diet . . . and the greater the need to accomplish this change.

Second, avoid foods that have excess salt when possible. Many snack foods and prepared foods have large amounts of salt. Many times the foods may not taste very salty even though the sodium content is very high. This does not mean you may *never* have any of these foods. You should simply avoid them when you have a choice. Did you know that some canned soups have more sodium than a person needs for a whole day? Table 33 lists common foods that are high in sodium. Try to avoid these when possible.

If you have questions about your diet, talk with your physician who can recommend a dietician to help in understanding your own dietary needs.

Weight Control.   High blood pressure and excess body weight (obesity) are related. Hypertension is more common in overweight persons. Persons who gain weight often notice that their blood pressure becomes higher as well. The reasons for this are not known, but it is important that if you are overweight you try to reduce. Many people find that their blood pressure becomes normal when they lose excess pounds. This is another way to treat hypertension without medication.

If you are overweight, you should try to reduce. Your desirable body weight depends on your height and build (see page 95). Check with your physician if you have questions.

Weight loss programs are discussed in Chapter 4. To lose weight, you must take in fewer calories than you use in your daily activity. There is no way to avoid this fact. For most people, success in weight loss depends on three conditions:

1. There is a strong commitment to lose weight. You must think it is important to lose weight—not just to please your spouse, friend, or family. Your feeling should be that "This is the time in my life I am going to lose weight, no matter what!"

2. Calorie intake is reduced. This can be done by following a restricted calorie diet as discussed in Chapter 4. These diets include a wide variety of foods. Another simple diet to follow is one in which you eat vegetables, salads, and meat at each meal but nothing else—no breads, potatoes, or desserts. This often allows a person to feel full but lose weight. This diet is also easy to follow when eating in restaurants.

3. A regular exercise program will allow you to use up more calories in a shorter time. An exercise program (discussed on pages 33–34) can begin with simply walking a short distance daily, gradually increasing the distance. Other benefits of an exercise program are a better control of appetite and an increase in the sense of well-being that comes with exercise. Before you start an exercise program, you should check with your physician.

If your weight loss is not successful then you should find out why. If there are no other medical problems present, you may need help in lowering your calorie intake. Suppressing your appetite with medication and using very low calorie liquid diet plans are other ways to accomplish weight loss. Long-term weight control is discussed further in Chapter 4. You should not give up if your efforts aren't quickly successful; it is only a matter of finding which weight loss program will work for you.

Start a Regular Exercise Program. A regular exercise program may also help lower blood pressure. Many exercise programs are available, including walking and bicycle riding. Choose an exercise that is convenient and that you enjoy (or at least don't mind). If you hate an exercise or it is not convenient, you probably will not continue it very long. If your schedule limits your free time, you may need to consider an exercise available at home such as an exercise bicycle. This would allow you to exercise at any time, regardless of weather and at your own convenience. Other exercises for busy people would be jumping rope, jogging, and swimming. These allow excellent exercise and can be effective in a short period of time. Try to exercise for 15–20 minutes a day, 5 days each week. Remember, before you start an exercise program, check with your physician to be sure that it is safe. Begin with very brief sessions of 1–2 minutes so that you are not tired or sore after the exercise.

Manage Your Stress.   Emotional stress and anxiety can raise blood pressure. Management of the stress due to job, family problems, and other personal problems can help control blood pressure. One way to manage stress is through a regular exercise program. Other ways include specific techniques to allow relaxation called the *relaxation response.* Your physician can give further specific suggestions to learn the relaxation response.

Lower Excess Alcohol Intake.   If you have hypertension and drink alcohol, you may find that lowering your intake of alcohol lowers blood pressure. Excess alcohol may cause an elevation in blood pressure, although the way this happens is not known. It is probably not necessary to stop alcohol completely to improve blood pressure in this situation. It has been recommended that alcohol be eliminated or at least reduced to the equivalent of no more than 24 ounces of beer or 8 ounces of wine or 1 ounce of 100 proof liquor each day. This alcohol intake guideline applies only to hypertension. Check with your physician to see if further limits are suggested in your own situation.

Potassium and Calcium Intake.   Researchers have found that lower levels of potassium intake may result in hypertension and increases in calcium intake in some persons may lower blood pressure.

The value of increased potassium or calcium intake in hypertension is not clear, however, very high intake of potassium or calcium may be dangerous. Until more information is available, it is recommended that you increase potassium or calcium in your diet or by supplement only under the direction of your physician.

Nontraditional Treatments in Hypertension

Some treatments are recommended by well-meaning persons, but they often have not been tested or have no proven value in lowering blood pressure. For example, certain plants and roots can be used in foods and teas; but until these remedies are tested, the effectiveness of such "potions" is not known. In fact, the side effects of these treatments is also unknown and, perhaps most important, the use of these treatments delays the start of effective treatment of hypertension. It is recommended that untested remedies be avoided, but if you feel strongly about trying one then talk with your physician for facts about that specific treatment.

Suggestion: If your blood pressure remains above 89 diastolic (lower number) or above 140 systolic (upper number) then specific actions are needed.

Treatment of Hypertension Using Medications

If treatment without medication does not lower blood pressure to the normal range then medications are available that can control blood pressure effectively with a minimum of side effects. If the diastolic blood pressure is lowered with treatment, there are fewer strokes, less heart failure, and fewer deaths. In some studies, a decrease in strokes by 30 to 50 percent has been found when hypertension is controlled.

When should medications be started in hypertension? This depends on your individual situation, but there are some guidelines:

1. First, try the methods outlined previously involving no medication including lowering your salt intake, controlling your body weight, maintaining a regular exercise program, decreasing alcohol intake, and managing stress.

2. If your diastolic blood pressure is still in the high normal range (85–89), check your blood pressure every 1 to 2 months.

3. If your diastolic blood pressure is still 90 to 94, treating with medications to lower the blood pressure to normal levels may be in order. Your physician might choose to watch the blood pressure closely and continue the treatments in 1. This decision could depend on whether you have other factors that increase the risk of cardiovascular disease, such as smoking cigarettes or high blood cholesterol.

4. If your diastolic blood pressure remains at 95 or greater, most physicians would consider adding medication to lower the blood pressure to normal levels. The methods outlined for treatment without medication should be continued as well. The choice of medications is discussed in the next section.

5. If your systolic blood pressure is above 160 then the methods outlined for treatment without medication should be continued. Many physicians would consider adding medication to lower your systolic blood pressure. The goal is to lower the blood pressure to 140 to 160 or

as close to this level as is reasonably possible without side effects from medicines.

6. If your diastolic blood pressure is 115 or greater then you should see your physician *immediately.*

Medications Available for Treatment in Hypertension

A large number of medications are available for the treatment of hypertension. For many years, diuretics were the first drugs given to begin treatment in most patients. These may be effective, are often able to be taken once daily, are usually well-tolerated, and are among the lower-priced of the medications used for hypertension.

Over the past 20 years many other medications have become available for the treatment of hypertension. A partial list of the medications currently available is shown in Table 3 on page 37.

Since there are so many choices available, the goals of treatment with medication are even more likely to be achieved—control of blood pressure with minimal side effects from medication and with a convenient dosage of medication. The newer medications may be more expensive.

If your blood pressure is not controlled within a reasonable time by the medication, your physician may choose to increase the dose of the same medication, another medication may be added, or the medication may be replaced by a different one. Treatment is individualized to give the best possible control of blood pressure with the fewest side effects. This may require some patience in order to find the proper combination of medications for your own situation.

Side Effects of Medications.   Almost every medicine has potential side effects. When any medication is taken, it should be for a specific purpose and side effects are *always* possible. If the potential benefits outweigh the possible side effects, the medication may be taken. The dangers of uncontrolled hypertension with future risk of stroke, heart attack, heart failure, and kidney disease are known. If these problems might be prevented with the help of a medication with minimal side effects, then it is a reasonable action to consider.

When you take a medication for hypertension you should have some idea of what it is expected to do, how long it might take to be effective, and what the potential side effects are.

Do not hesitate to report side effects. Many problems may not be related to the medication, but your physician needs to know about *any* changes you experience when taking medication. If the new

TABLE 3
Hypertension Medications*

Diuretics	Adrenergic Inhibitors (cont.)
Bendroflumethiazide (Naturetin)	Timolol (Blocadren)
Chlorthiazide (Diuril)	Clonidine (Catapres)
Chlothalidone (Hygroton)	Guanabenz (Wytensin)
Hydrochlorthiazide (Esidrix, Hydrodiuril)	Methlydopa (Aldomet)
Indapamide (Lozol)	Prazosin (Minipres)
Methyclothiazde (Diulo, Zaroxolyn)	Labetalol (Normodyne)
Trichlormethiazide (Naqua)	
Bumetanide (Bumex)	*Vasodilators*
Ethacrynic acid (Edacrin)	Hydralazine (Apresoline)
Furosemide (Lasix)	Minoxidil (Loniten)
Amiloride (Midamor)	
Spironolactone (Aldactone)	*Angiotensin Converting Enzyme Inhibitors*
Triamterene (Dyrenium)	
(combinations of more than one are available)	Captopril (Capoten)
	Enalapril (Vasotec)
	Lisinopril (Prinivil)
Adrenergic Inhibitors	*Calcium Channel Blockers*
Atenolol (Tenormin)	
Metoprolol (Lopressor)	Diltiazem (Cardizem)
Nadolol (Corgard)	Nifedipine (Procardia)
Pindolol (Visken)	Verapimil (Calan, Isoptin)
Propranolol (Inderal)	

*Many other medications are available which may be given by mouth or by injection. Choice of medications depends on other medical problems present, preference because of side effects, convenience, and expense. Your physician can help you find the best choice for you.

problem is caused by the medication, it will need to be resolved. This can be done by changing the dose of medication, changing to another medication, or correcting the problem in another way.

There is some power of suggestion possible when side effects are discussed, especially when we are told that feelings such as fatigue and weakness may happen. These feelings very commonly have causes other than medication. However, all *new* feelings and signs should be reported, especially if they start after beginning a medication.

Be honest with your physician. If you have *any* questions or concerns about the steps you are taking to control hypertension then you need more information. In treating any type of health concern effectively, it is vital that you and your physician establish a relationship with open communication. Use Checklist 1 if you have high blood pressure.

CHECKLIST 1
BLOOD PRESSURE

Systolic (Upper) Blood Pressure

Less than 140	Recheck yearly
140–159	Recheck within 2 months
Over 159	Needs evaluation within 2 weeks

Diastolic (Lower) Blood Pressure

Less than 85	Recheck within 2 years
85–89	Recheck within 1 year
90–104	See your physician
105–114	Needs evaluation within 2 weeks
Over 114	Needs immediate medical care

Date	Time	Blood Pressure
_____	_____	_____
_____	_____	_____
_____	_____	_____
_____	_____	_____
_____	_____	_____
_____	_____	_____

Medication name: _____

Directions: _____

Pharmacy number: _____

Questions, feelings, side effects:

Date: _____

Date: _____

Date: _____

Date: _____

Once normal, your blood pressure should be measured regularly to be sure good control is maintained. Measurements might be weekly at first, then less often if normal. Your physician can tell you how often you should be seen to be sure side effects are not a problem. Blood tests may be needed occasionally when taking some medications.

Be prepared to continue medications for hypertension over a long period of time. After one year of normal blood pressure it may be possible to lower or stop medication but *only under the direction of your physician*. Do not stop your medication without talking with your physician.

Do not run out of medicine. Keep a supply at home and refill the prescription *before* you run out. Your blood pressure may rise quickly and other serious problems may occur if medications are suddenly stopped.

Suggestion: Using treatment without medication and medications when needed, blood pressure can be maintained at normal levels to prevent future disease.

■ HIGH BLOOD CHOLESTEROL LEVELS

Cholesterol is normally present in the blood. If the blood level of cholesterol is elevated, the risk is greater for atherosclerosis, especially in the coronary arteries that supply blood to the heart. The higher the level of cholesterol, the higher the risk becomes. The exact way in which this high cholesterol level causes atherosclerosis to progress more rapidly is not known.

Lowering elevated cholesterol levels reduces the risk of later development of coronary heart disease. It seems reasonable to expect that atherosclerosis in other blood vessels would also be prevented or delayed, but there is less definite evidence of this. However, the evidence is extremely strong that there should be a maximum effort to control abnormal blood cholesterol levels.

What level of cholesterol is too high? For many years, the "normal" level of cholesterol was thought to be up to around 300 mg/dl. In 1985, a group of researchers presented some guidelines (Table 4) to allow a better understanding of what "high cholesterol" should mean. These levels are now widely accepted and are used to help guide diet and other treatment. In brief:

< 200 mg/dl	Desirable
200–239 mg/dl	Borderline high blood cholesterol
240 mg/dl or greater	High blood cholesterol

TABLE 4
Coronary Risk Profile*

Determination:	Result:
Cholesterol	271 mg/dl
Triglycerides	249 mg/dl
HDL cholesterol	26 mg/dl
LDL cholesterol	194 mg/dl
VLDL cholesterol	51 mg/dl
Cholesterol/HDL ratio	10.4

	Desirable	Borderline/high	High
Total cholesterol	<200	200–239	240 or more
Total triglycerides	<250	250–499	500 or more
HDL cholesterol	50 or more	36–49	35 or less
LDL cholesterol	<130	130–159	160 or more
VLDL cholesterol	20 or less	21–39	40 or more

CHOL/HDL-C Ratio	Half Average	Average	2X Average	3X Average
Male	3.43	4.97	9.55	23.99
Female	3.27	4.44	7.05	11.04

*This person was found to have high blood cholesterol. LDL-Cholesterol is high. HDL-Cholesterol is low. The Cholesterol/HDL ratio suggest a risk over 2 times average for coronary heart disease.

These guidelines are for cholesterol measured as total cholesterol. The laboratory measurements can be confusing because results can be described in several different ways. Cholesterol and other fats (lipids) do not circulate in the blood alone, but are carried by a protein. The protein which is most associated with cholesterol is low density lipoprotein (LDL). The higher the LDL-cholesterol levels, the higher the risk of coronary heart disease.

There are other proteins in the blood which carry fats, including one called high density lipoprotein (HDL), a protein which in part carries cholesterol but has been found to have a beneficial effect. In fact, studies have shown that the *higher* the levels of HDL, the lower the risk of coronary heart disease. The exact reasons for this protective effect are not yet known. HDL-cholesterol has been called the "good" cholesterol.

Very low density lipoprotein (VLDL) also carries a portion of the total blood cholesterol. Another type of fat or lipid in the blood is called *triglyceride*. Triglycerides are associated with the protein VLDL when circulating in the blood.

When measuring cholesterol levels, you may receive several different laboratory results including total cholesterol, LDL-cholesterol, HDL-cholesterol, VLDL-cholesterol, and triglycerides. (See Table 7)

The risk of coronary heart disease and death rises along with the total blood cholesterol level and the LDL-cholesterol level. For example, a person whose total cholesterol level is 240 mg/dl has twice the risk of a level of 200 mg/dl for coronary heart disease and death. Lowering the cholesterol level reduces the chance of further worsening of coronary heart disease in those persons who already have the disease. In persons who have hypertension or who smoke, this effect is even greater in lowering the chance of disease. For example, a person who has a high blood cholesterol level along with hypertension and who smokes cigarettes may have 4 to 5 times the risk of heart disease and death compared to the person with only high blood cholesterol.

These terms and numbers can be confusing, but there are some simple guidelines. To detect high blood cholesterol, a blood test is needed. The NCEP suggests measurements in all adults over age 20 at least once every 5 years. This simple blood test is easily available and can be done at any time of day without fasting. We also recommend after age 30 to 35 that the level be checked every 1 to 2 years if it remains "desirable." Other risk factors as shown on page 28 should be looked for as well. These should be removed or controlled. You should follow the general guidelines for a diet to limit cholesterol as shown on page 97.

If your total cholesterol is 200 mg/dl or greater then the test should be repeated within 8 weeks. If still abnormal, if you already have coronary heart disease, or if you have other risk factors then LDL-cholesterol is also measured to decide if further action is needed. Recommendations for levels of LDL-cholesterol in adults are suggested by the National Cholesterol Education Project (NCEP):

Desirable LDL-cholesterol	130 mg/dl
Borderline LDL-cholesterol	130–159 mg/dl
High LDL-cholesterol	160 mg/dl or greater

LDL-cholesterol is measured after fasting for 12 hours (for example, nothing to eat or drink except water overnight). If your results show borderline high LDL-cholesterol or high LDL-cholesterol then your physician can guide further treatment. This treatment should include a specific diet to lower cholesterol as well as remove other risk factors such as smoking cigarettes, excess body weight, and lack of a regular exercise program.

HDL-cholesterol is usually measured when LDL-cholesterol is measured. Some laboratories report the ratio of total cholesterol to HDL-cholesterol. A ratio of 4.5 to 4.9 is an average risk of coronary heart disease. A ratio of 3.3 is about 1/2 average risk (see Table 7). If HDL-cholesterol is found to be low, it seems reasonable to try to raise the HDL-cholesterol level since this may lower the risk of coronary heart disease. It is interesting that what raises the HDL-cholesterol is a recommended practice anyway. The following prescription for raising HDL-cholesterol is encouraged:

Some Ways to Raise HDL-Cholesterol (Beneficial)

- Control your body weight
- Add a regular exercise program
- Stop cigarettes
- Some medications used to lower LDL-cholesterol may raise HDL-cholesterol

Triglycerides are the other major fat that is commonly measured in the blood. Abnormally high triglycerides alone have not been shown to be as important as cholesterol for prevention of heart disease. Levels less than 250 mg/dl are considered normal. Levels of 250 to 500 mg/dl are considered borderline elevated and levels of greater than 500 mg/dl are considered high. In many cases, the levels of triglycerides will decrease as other risk factors are controlled. These include controlling your weight, adding a regular exercise program, and lowering your cholesterol level to normal with diet. Triglyceride levels should be measured fasting. If your triglyceride results are 250 mg/dl or greater, then talk with your physician. Then planning can be done depending on your other risk factors and other medical problems.

With the knowledge of your blood cholesterol and triglyceride levels, you can begin to manage your future health. If the levels are "borderline" or "high" it is important to talk to your physician. There are certain other medical problems that can cause high cholesterol or high triglyceride levels. In these cases, the underlying problem must be discovered and treated. If no other causes are found, then usual treatment would include a specific *diet* to lower cholesterol or triglycerides, *weight loss* if you are overweight, and a *regular exercise program*. Medictions may be needed.

Diet is essential and has been shown to be effective in lowering levels of cholesterol and triglycerides. These diets are discussed in Chapter 5.

It may take up to 6 months for your diet to lower the level of LDL-cholesterol. The goal of diet is to lower LDL-cholesterol to less than 160 mg/dl (or total cholesterol to less than 240 mg/dl) if you have no other risk factors and you do not have coronary heart disease already. If you already have coronary heart disease or if you have other risk factors then the LDL-cholesterol levels should be lowered to less than 130 mg/dl (or total cholesterol of less than 200 mg/dl).

A *regular exercise program* helps in weight loss and increases the level of HDL. HDL levels in long distance runners and other athletes have been found to be higher than those who do not exercise. Ask your physician before you begin an exercise program, since other risk factors and other medical problems will affect what level of exercise is safe for you. A goal of 20 to 40 minutes of exercise 3 to 5 times each week is reasonable (see p. 33).

If these measures are not successful over a period of 6 months, a number of *medications are available* for treatment to lower abnormal blood cholesterol and triglyceride levels. In some severe cases, medications may be started earlier than 6 months or along with a specific diet. Many medications are available, including some with minimal side effects. These medications usually require several months to show their effect on cholesterol levels. They should be taken in combination with a proper diet, attempts to control excess weight, and a regular exercise program.

Some of the Medications Most Commonly Used to Treat High Blood Cholesterol

Cholestyramine	(Questran)
Cholestipol	(Colestid)
Clofibrate	(Atromid-S)
Gemfibrozil	(Lopid)
Lovastatin	(Mevacor)
Nicotinic Acid	(Niacin, Lipo-Nicin, Nicobid, Nico-400, Nicolar Tablets)

It is necessary to have blood tests after you begin medication to be sure that it is actually lowering the blood cholesterol and to be sure that no unwanted effects happen. Blood tests to measure the levels of total cholesterol or LDL-cholesterol may be needed at intervals of 3 or 4 months until the levels are normal. Then less frequent testing will monitor your levels. When these blood tests are taken, tests can also be done to help identify side effects. You should be aware of any potential side effects if you are taking a medication. Your physician can guide you in this, depending on which medicine is used.

Fish products, especially fish oil, may lower cholesterol levels. Eskimos, for example, have a low amount of atherosclerosis and they follow a diet high in fish products. These diets usually contain more protein, less saturated fat, and more polyunsaturated fat than many Western diets. Researchers have found that it would be necessary to eat fairly large amounts of certain fish or fish oil to affect cholesterol and triglyceride levels. However, a diet that contains larger amounts of fish would generally be healthier than a diet rich in red meat. Taking large amounts of fish oil or marine products to lower cholesterol levels is still considered to be in the testing phase by most researchers. This would be recommended only if advised by your physician. Remember that fish products fried or salted may lose much of their advantage because of the fat and salt content.

Should we all be on a low cholesterol diet? The answer would appear to be yes. The actual causes of atherosclerosis are still not known. It takes many years for atherosclerosis to develop; therefore, it is reasonable to think (but not yet proven) that a diet low in cholesterol might delay the development of atherosclerosis. The facts will probably not be known for a number of years. At that point, you may find that you should have followed a low cholesterol diet for the previous 10 or 20 years! A reasonable solution is to follow a prudent diet, moderate in cholesterol—not over 300 mg each day. This diet is discussed in Chapter 5. Your success in controlling this part of your health can make a direct difference in the length and quality of your life. But remember, there are no early symptoms or signs.

Suggestion: Measure your total blood cholesterol yearly. If above 200 mg/dl, specific action is needed.

■ CIGARETTE SMOKING

Cigarette smoking is another major risk factor for coronary heart disease. It has been estimated that 300,000 deaths in the United States each year are tobacco-related. Today about 50 million people in the United States smoke. Smoking is a major risk factor for atherosclerosis and greatly increases the risk of coronary heart disease, atherosclerosis in the arteries of the legs, and atherosclerosis in the arteries that supply the brain. Think of the reduction of these diseases if smoking were stopped!

A list of some of the other major diseases and medical problems that have been linked to smoking follows. These are discussed in other chapters as well. Each of these problems gives an excellent reason to stop smoking.

Let's review some of the facts about smoking as a risk factor and then review some specific suggestions that may help you stop this deadly habit. Once smokers understand the medical consequences for themselves and others, it becomes easier to quit. Excellent support is available during the difficult period of withdrawal.

Some Medical Problems Due to Cigarette Smoking

A report of the Smoking Education Program of the National Institute of Health reviewed the areas of increased risk caused by smoking:

- Coronary heart disease, especially heart attack, heart failure
- Magnifies the risk for coronary heart disease in those who already have higher risk from hypertension and high blood cholesterol
- Atherosclerosis and blockage of the arteries that supply the legs—leading to gangrene and amputation
- Atherosclerosis and blockage of the arteries that supply the brain—leading to stroke
- Increased risk of sudden death
- Coronary heart disease and stroke in women who take oral contraceptives (especially after age 35)
- Peptic ulcers and may interfere with the treatment of the ulcer disease
- Cancer in the mouth, throat (larynx), esophagus, lung, kidney, bladder, and pancreas
- Blood cholesterol increased by increasing LDL-cholesterol and may decrease HDL-cholesterol
- Emphysema and chronic bronchitis (chronic lung disease)
- Cough, respiratory infections, and asthma illnesses
- Physical performance, endurance, and lung function decreased

- Respiratory infection in infants whose parents smoke
- Miscarriage, stillbirth, and low birth weight of the infant
- May interfere with the action of medications given for other medical problems

Benefits of Stopping Cigarette Smoking

- Decreases the risk of coronary heart disease including decreasing the death rate. It has been estimated that 10 years after stopping smoking, a person who smoked less than 1 pack per day has about the same death rate as a person who never smoked.
- Decreases the risk of death after a heart attack, coronary bypass surgery, and other surgery
- Decreases the risk of atherosclerosis and blockage of the arteries in the legs
- Improves physical endurance
- Improves the chance of effective treatment of peptic ulcer
- Lowers the risk of miscarriage and other pregnancy-related problems
- Lowers the risk of cancer in the mouth, throat (larynx), esophagus, lung, kidney, bladder, and pancreas.

The facts are clear that smoking is deadly; it is one factor that *can be* controlled. Make a commitment: This is the time in my life when I will finally stop smoking.

Once you have taken these important steps, realize that much help and support is available. Contact your local chapter of the American Lung Association or the American Cancer Society. They can help you make contact with local programs. Talk with your physician who can also guide you to other sources of support. Choose a reputable smoking withdrawal clinic, if necessary. Decide that you will find whatever way is necessary to stop smoking.

Many people feel actual withdrawal symptoms from the stoppage of nicotine. These symptoms may be severe, especially in heavy smokers. These feelings usually last 1 or 2 weeks, then disappear. After that, the actual physical withdrawal should not remain a problem, although the urge to smoke may return. It is this 1- or 2-week period in which support from family, friends, and your physician can be very helpful. The newer nicotine chewing gum may allow a person to reduce the feelings of withdrawal. The gum is used to avoid the withdrawal symptoms, then it is gradually eliminated.

It will help to be aware of what feelings you might have during this period of withdrawal. Some people have little difficulty in quitting the habit. Others are not quite as lucky.

Suggestion: The evidence to stop smoking for medical reasons is overwhelming. Make your commitment now to stop smoking.

■ A REGULAR EXERCISE PROGRAM

People who have a regular exercise program have a lower risk of developing coronary heart disease than persons who are inactive. This is difficult to prove because it is difficult to separate the effect of exercise from other daily habits such as diet and cigarette use. Exercise, as discussed earlier, can be helpful for weight control and relaxation as well. Regular exercise may raise HDL-cholesterol levels, which is one factor that may lower the risk of coronary heart disease (see p. 33).

Suggestion: A regular exercise program is an important part of the removal of a risk factor for atherosclerosis.

■ EXCESS BODY WEIGHT (OBESITY)

Statistics show that being overweight (obese) increases your risk of coronary heart disease. The more overweight you are, the greater the risk of death from coronary heart disease as well as other causes. The exact reasons for the increased risk of heart disease are not known. Obesity increases the risk of hypertension, high blood cholesterol, and other problems which may help explain the higher risk.

Suggestion: Maintaining desirable body weight is an important part of the control of the risk factor for atherosclerosis (see page 209).

■ STRESS MANAGEMENT FOR HOSTILITY AND ANGER

Certain patterns of behavior can increase the risk of coronary heart disease. The most important behavior pattern so far has been called Type A. These people can often be recognized by the following behaviors:

- Impatient
- Very competitive
- Hurried
- Strong desire for achievement
- Aggression that may be held back or repressed

Type A behavior is thought to be a result of a combination of personality and past experiences. Type B behavior patterns are more relaxed, easy going, and less hurried, with a lower risk of coronary heart disease.

The most important aspects of the Type A behavior pattern related to heart disease are hostility and anger. These both seem to be the main factors that in some way cause the risk to increase. Both hostility and anger may also cause an increase in feelings of stress and anxiety.

It is not necessary to be a Type A personality to be productive or to achieve high goals in life. Those with Type B behavior may have the same level of motivation, work, and productivity as those with Type A behavior. Type B behavior can allow a better sense of inner security to be productive without the need to compete and with less fear of failure.

Other stress and anxiety may contribute to hypertension, over-eating, and limited activity and exercise. These problems may increase the risk of coronary heart disease. Stress is a normal part of our lives and is not always bad. Stress can lead us to take actions that often improve our lives. For example, anxiety and stress caused by the discovery of high blood cholesterol may lead us to follow a diet, exercise, and lose weight, thus lowering the blood cholesterol and reducing the risk of heart disease.

If you feel an uncomfortable amount of hostility, anger, or other anxiety, you should consider asking your physician for advice. Being aware of this source of stress can help you take action to manage the stress more effectively. Stress management techniques are available. One technique, called the *relaxation response*, is easily learned. You can learn these and other steps to take to control anxiety and stress without making major changes in your life.

■ CONTROL OF DIABETES MELLITUS

Diabetics (those persons who have diabetes mellitus) suffer from a problem in which the level of blood glucose is abnormally high.

Persons who have this problem are at greater risk for coronary heart disease for reasons that are not known. A blood test which can tell if the blood glucose is high is done in many routine examinations. If your blood glucose is high, you definitely should see your physician for further information and possible treatment including diet and other measures. The blood glucose should be maintained as close to normal levels as possible. It is very important that other risk factors for coronary heart disease be controlled or removed as well. See page 179 for more discussion of diabetes mellitus.

Suggestion: Control of diabetes mellitus is an important part of the control of risk factors for atherosclerosis.

■ DOES ASPIRIN HELP?

Over the years, it has been found that aspirin used in low doses, even less than one each day, changes the action of blood platelets. Platelets are important in forming a blood clot. Platelets may also be involved in the process of atherosclerosis, including the hardening and narrowing of arteries in the heart, brain, and other organs.

The low dose of aspirin changes the way platelets work in a way that may help prevent unwanted blood clots. Many people can tolerate a low dose of aspirin with few or no side effects. Talk with your physician to see if such a plan might be useful in your own situation. Since everyone is different and there are potential side effects, do not start the aspirin technique until you check with your physician.

■ RISK FACTORS WHICH CANNOT BE CHANGED

Family History of Premature Coronary Heart Disease. Heart attacks or other forms of coronary heart disease before age 50 are called premature coronary heart disease. If you have a family member who suffered from premature coronary heart disease, your own risk is also increased. This risk factor can't be removed but it may be managed. If other risk factors, especially hypertension, high blood cholesterol, or smoking are present, you should make every effort to reduce them.

Suggestion: If your family has 1 or more members affected by coronary heart disease before age 50, you should take extra effort to control and remove your other risk factors. This will reduce your risk of coronary heart disease to the lowest possible level.

Age.   Another risk factor for coronary heart disease that we can't control is age. The older we get, the higher the risk of coronary heart disease. However, many older persons do not develop coronary heart disease. Some areas of the world have much less disease at older ages. It is important that we focus on those risk factors that we can control and remove in order to lower our overall risk of coronary heart disease.

Sex.   Men are at much greater risk for coronary heart disease than women until the age of menopause in women (45–55). After menopause, the risk increases in women.

All of the causes for this difference are not known. The female hormone estrogen may help protect and lower the risk in younger women. At menopause, the level of estrogen decreases, the menstrual periods stop, and the risk of coronary heart disease increases. It is thought that other causes are also present, but they are not known at this time.

Suggestion: Men can't control this risk factor, but other risk factors which can be controlled and removed should be emphasized. Women should be aware that after menopause their own risk of coronary heart disease increases and other risk factors must be controlled.

Once the risks are identified, you can begin to control or remove each risk factor. Remember that it does not require a great deal of time in your physician's office or clinic and it should not require a great deal of your own time to actually control these risk factors. The benefits of lowering your risk of heart attack and other disease are overwhelming compared to the small amount of time spent removing risk factors. If you have a heart attack and if you survive then your life will change greatly. You will then spend a great deal of your time and effort controlling risk factors to prevent further heart attacks. Why not spend much less time and effort earlier to prevent or delay this disease if possible?

Talk with your physician. Look at the guidelines on page 28 for suggestions to easily and effectively identify your own risk factors for coronary heart disease and other atherosclerosis.

■ IDENTIFY AND REMOVE YOUR RISK FACTORS FOR CANCER

Based on medical statistics, it has been estimated that about one-third of all Americans will develop a malignancy (cancer) in their lifetime.

At least one-half of these persons will die from their malignancy. To improve these statistics, efforts need to be made to prevent the development of malignant diseases. An example of identifying and removing a causative agent (carcinogen) is stopping cigarette smoking to prevent later development of lung cancer.

It is difficult to identify the agents that cause cancer. Cancer rarely develops after a single exposure to a carcinogen. It usually requires many exposures over long periods of time and it is usually many years after exposure before the cancer becomes apparent. Cancer does not develop in all persons exposed to the causative agent. Once a possible cause is identified and removed, it takes many years to appreciate a decrease in the cancer caused by that agent. For example, the risk of lung cancer is directly related to smoke exposure. It is rare to develop cancer in less than 20 years of smoking, and all smokers do not develop lung cancer. It takes 7 to 10 years after stopping smoking to notice a reduction in the risk of lung cancer.

Risk factors can be identified which clearly increase the chance of certain cancers. Avoiding these factors is recommended to lessen the risk of developing a malignant disease. Let's look at some of these risk factors.

Smoking.   While there has been significant political and legal controversy regarding the relationship of tobacco products to cancer, the vast majority of the medical literature suggests a clear relationship between smoking cigarettes and later development of cancer. Compared to a nonsmoker, smokers have about 10 times the risk of developing lung cancer. The risk of cancer of the larynx, mouth, throat, esophagus, bladder, and pancreas are also greatly increased. Likewise, smoking has been related to other diseases such as lung disease and heart disease. It is difficult to estimate the billions of dollars spent yearly on tobacco-related illnesses. The recommendations of medical evidence and the American Cancer Society are to avoid the use of all tobacco products.

Alcohol.   Alcohol has not been shown to be a direct cause of cancer. However, alcohol in combination with tobacco use increases the risk of developing cancer in the mouth, throat, larynx, and esophagus, compared to nondrinking smokers and compared to nonsmokers. If you use alcoholic beverages, it is recommended that you do so in moderation and that you avoid exposure to tobacco products.

Radiation.   Radiation increases the risk of developing cancer in direct proportion to the amount of radiation received. There is an increase in various malignancies in radiologists (physicians specializing in the use of x-ray testing) who don't use proper protective shielding. There is also increased risk of cancer in persons who receive radiation for benign diseases, atomic bomb survivors, and even in long-term cancer survivors who received treatment with radiation. While the dose of radiation received from diagnostic x-rays is usually quite low, it is recommended that any unnecessary x-rays be avoided.

Chemicals.   Many industrial and medical chemicals have been identified as carcinogens. When this is discovered, the industrial agents are usually removed from general use. Generally, the medical agents are only used in individuals with severe life-threatening illnesses in whom other treatments have failed.

Hormone Treatment.   The use of the female hormone estrogen has been associated with an increased risk of developing cancer of the lining of the uterus (endometrial cancer). However, the evidence that synthetic estrogens may protect against development of osteoporosis has caused resurgence in the use of estrogens. Discuss the benefits and risks of estrogen treatment with your physician before starting any sort of long-term use. This is discussed on page 55.

Sunlight.   Sunlight has been shown to increase the risk of developing basal cell and squamous cell cancers of the skin. If treated early, this cancer is rarely fatal though they can be deforming. It is controversial whether sunlight increases the risk of developing the other most common type of skin cancer, malignant melanoma (cancerous mole). Regardless, one should avoid excessive exposure to sunlight by use of clothing or sunscreen. This is discussed on page 218.

Diet.   The effect of diet on the subsequent development of malignancy is hard to document. Medical researchers compare the relative risk of developing malignancy in societies with the different dietary habits. Using these epidemiologic studies, the American Cancer Society recommends that individuals avoid obesity; decrease total fat intake; eat more high-fiber foods such as whole grain cereals, fruits, and vegetables; include foods rich in vitamins A and C; include cruciferous vegetables such as cabbage, broccoli, brussel sprouts, and cauliflower; and be moderate in the consumption of salt-cured, smoked, and nitrite-cured foods. This is discussed on page 113.

■ DETECT CANCER EARLY

Over the years medical statistics have shown that the earlier cancer is detected and appropriate treatment begun, the less likely the disease will be fatal. It is not possible to screen everyone for all malignancies. A screening test must be reliable, relatively simple, cost effective, and relatively harmless. Screening for early detection of many of the most common kinds of cancer is available.

CHECKLIST 2
EARLY CANCER DETECTION

Women

Breast examination by a physician	Every 2–3 years up to age 40, then yearly
Pelvic examination	Every 2 years after age 20 until age 40, then yearly
Pap test	By age 18, then every 2 years until age 70, then every 3 years
Mammogram (a type of x-ray of the breast)	By age 38, then every 2 years to age 50, then yearly

Men and Women

Rectal examination	By age 30, then at age 35, age 40, then yearly
Stool test for blood	At age 40, then yearly
Sigmoidoscopy (direct examination of the rectum and adjacent area of the lower intestine)	Recommended by some experts at age 50, then every 5 years. Some persons may need this more or less often. Ask your physician for advice on your own situation
Skin changes	Watch your skin for new moles or old ones which change. If any area of skin becomes darker, new or old moles enlarge or bleed or become painful, see your physician
Mouth & throat changes	Report any sores or color changes in your mouth which persist or are painful. This is especially important for persons who use *any* form of tobacco

Others

Eye examination	Every 2 years
Dental examination	Yearly

Breast Cancer in Women. Self-examination of the breast, breast examination by a physician, and mammography have been shown to identify early breast cancers with improved survival. It is recommended that women perform a self-examination of each breast every month. Breast examination by a physician is recommended every 2–3 years up to age 40, then yearly. A baseline mammogram is recommended around age 38, then every other year from ages 40 to 50, then yearly.

Pelvic Cancer in Women. All women should have a pelvic examination every 2 years after age 20 until age 40, then yearly. A Pap test is recommended by age 18, then every 2 years until age 70, then every 3 years. In some cases the Pap test may be performed less frequently if there have been several normal tests depending on the individual situation. If the Pap test is abnormal, there may be more frequent testing. A sample of the uterine endometrial tissue may be recommended at menopause in certain persons.

These tests can detect the three most common cancers of the pelvis—cancer of the cervix, cancer of the uterus, cancer of the ovary—as well as others.

Colon and Rectal Cancer. It is recommended that all persons have a rectal exam by age 30, then at age 35, at age 40, then yearly. The stool test for blood should also be obtained by age 40, then yearly. Sigmoidoscopy (direct examination of the rectum and adjacent area of the lower intestine) is recommended by many experts at age 50 then every 3–5 years depending on your individual situation.

Lung Cancer. Unfortunately, chest x-rays have not been shown to be very effective in early detection of lung cancer. Most effective is the avoidance of smoking cigarettes. Your physician can guide you to your own need for chest x-ray.

Skin Cancer. Watch for new moles or old ones that change. If any area of skin becomes darker, moles enlarge, bleed or become painful then you should see your physician. For those who have many moles it may be useful to see your physician or dermatologist on a yearly basis for your protection.

Mouth and Throat Cancer. Report any sores or color changes in your mouth which persist or are painful. If any hoarseness persists for 2 weeks then see your physician. These guidelines are especially important for persons who use *any* form of tobacco.

Checklist 2 summarizes these early cancer detection techniques.

■ IDENTIFY AND REMOVE YOUR RISK FACTORS FOR OSTEOPOROSIS

Osteoporosis means a decrease in the density of bone—thinning of the bones. As bones become thinner, they become easier to break. Minor injuries may then result in a broken bone. Eventually, even usual daily activities such as bending and walking can result in a fracture. The problem is that the bones that are commonly involved are those that allow us to be active—spine, hip, wrist, shoulder, pelvis, and feet (Figure 6).

Most persons first find out about osteoporosis when they suffer a fracture. A hip is broken or a bone in the spine is fractured and the x-ray reveals osteoporosis that has most likely been present and gradually worsening over a number of years.

There is no single specific cause of osteoporosis. It seems likely that there are many factors that contribute to the disease. Some persons are much more likely to develop osteoporosis than others. There are certain risk factors that greatly increase the risk of osteoporosis (Table 5). Many of these risk factors are treatable especially if identified early. With proper prevention and treatment the risk of broken bones and crippling also decreases.

Even if risk factors are not removed at an early age, osteoporosis can be detected early enough to plan treatment to prevent future

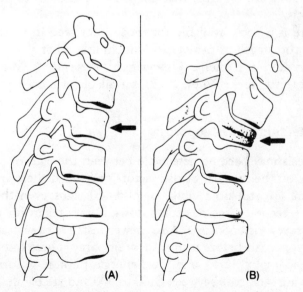

FIGURE 6   (A) Normal spine. (B) Spine with compression fracture. Note shortening of vertebra and abnormal curve of spine.

TABLE 5
Risk Factors for Osteoporosis

1. Lack of regular exercise program
2. Menopause in women, especially early menopause
3. Age 40 or older
4. Female sex
5. White race
6. Cigarette smoking
7. Family members who have osteoporosis
8. Underweight for your height
9. Heavy alcohol use
10. Certain medications: Cortisone-like drugs
11. Certain medical problems:
    Rheumatoid arthritis
    Emphysema, chronic bronchitis
    Hyperthyroidism
    Some types of stomach surgery
    Diabetes mellitus
    Other uncommon problems
12. Low calcium in diet

fractures. Tests are available that are sensitive enough to detect early osteoporosis.

There is a book available for those interested in further explanation of the stages of osteoporosis including what you can do for prevention and treatment. *Osteoporosis: Prevention, Management, Treatment* (New York: Wiley, 1988) is available at most bookstores.

Early Detection of Osteoporosis

Osteoporosis may become detectable between the ages of 35 and 55, depending on the number of risk factors present. If there are no fractures, there are still no feelings or outward signs even though this may be the second stage of osteoporosis. X-rays taken for other reasons may reveal osteoporosis. Also, newer tests are now available that detect osteoporosis before it may show on x-ray. These tests are computed tomography (CT) and dual-energy photon absorptiometry. Both tests are safe, cost between $100 to 300 and are painless. Neither test can tell definitely whether a person will have a fracture in the future, but it may give your physician useful information, especially if other treatments for osteoporosis are under consideration.

If osteoporosis is detected or if there has been a fracture and the osteoporosis is definitely present, then several steps should be considered.

1. Remove all risk factors possible as discussed previously.
2. Begin a regular exercise program as guided by your physician.
3. Consider whether to add estrogen in women after menopause on the advice of your physician.
4. Be sure of 1,500 mg calcium intake daily.
5. Other medications are available for treatment of osteoporosis. These include vitamin D which helps increase the body's absorption of calcium as well as medications including fluoride and calcitonin. The use of vitamin D and these medications should be under the supervision of your physician.

Suggestion: Specific measures are needed for treatment in order to prevent further fractures if osteoporosis is detectable.

■ SUMMARY

Once you know the risk factors for the major problems that may affect you as you mature, you can take specific steps to eliminate those over which you have control. With early prevention and detection of disease when treatment is most effective, you can approach the mature years with greater confidence.

CHAPTER 3

The Routine Medical Exam

As discussed earlier, detection of a physical problem is one of the keys to continuing good health. The personal examination by your physician including a discussion of history, feelings, and problems along with physical examination is still the most effective way to detect many medical problems.

Certain medical problems are much more likely to occur at certain ages in men and women. Instead of a yearly checkup that includes the same tests for all persons, it is much more effective to have a plan for each individual. This will allow early detection of problems that will most likely occur with the least amount of time and expense. This individualized plan is usually even more effective in finding important problems, but requires less time than many older "yearly" complete physical examinations.

For example, breast cancer is the most common cancer in women. Early detection allows treatment when it is most effective and may cure this cancer. Women can achieve early detection by learning self-examination of the breast and by having mammograms at certain times. Since breast cancer occurs in women especially after age 40, these are the years especially important for detection.

Still another example is a type of skin cancer, melanoma. Until a few years ago this was usually a fatal disease. Now persons at higher risk (including those who are fair-skinned and frequently exposed to sunlight over years) can know the facts. If these skin changes are found early, the disease is curable just by removal of the melanoma.

■ GOALS OF THE ROUTINE MEDICAL EXAM

The goals of a routine health exam are:

1. Detect risk factors that can be controlled or removed to prevent other diseases.
2. Detect certain specific problems early when easily treated to prevent more serious disease later.

As discussed in Chapter 1, it is not possible to do every test on all persons each year to detect disease. But certain tests give excellent results in finding risk factors and other diseases. All experts do not agree exactly on how often each test should be done. Some suggest more frequent tests than others. Each plan tries to find the most problems with the least trouble and expense. For further details and discussion of the choices choose a reference on page 307. Remember, each person is different. Talk with your physician to see which plan would be best for you.

■ STEP ONE: A COMPLETE MEDICAL HISTORY

At some point after age 18 you should have a complete history and physical examination by your physician. At this time, a complete record of your past illnesses and medical history is begun and a physical examination is completed. This will usually include the items in the medical history Checklist 3. Remember that this record will be available in the future if you are seen by another physician.

If all tests are normal, this history and physical examination should be repeated at age 30 and about every 5 years until age 50. Then decide with your physician how often to repeat the full exam.

If medical problems are found, your physician can help you decide what other steps are needed for proper diagnosis and treatment. Specific follow-up care can be planned as necessary.

History And Physical Examination

A complete health history and physical examination is recommended beginning sometime after age 18. Repeat again at around age 30. Then repeat about every 5 years until age 50. Then repeat yearly or as often as suggested by your physician. This visit will usually include most of the following items:

CHECKLIST 3
MEDICAL HISTORY

50-Year-Old Man[1]   *Last Date Completed*

1. A. Complete medical history and physical
   examination   _____

   B. Laboratory including blood cholesterol,
   glucose, urinalysis, and others if needed   _____

2. Risk factor review for coronary heart disease
   (Table _____)   _____

3. Early cancer detection (Checklist 3)   _____

4. Eye exam if not in past 2 years   _____

5. Dental exam if not in past year   _____

6. Review immunizations (p. _____)   _____

50-Year-Old Woman[2]   *Last Date Completed*

1. A. Complete medical history and physical
   examination   _____

   B. Laboratory including blood cholesterol,
   glucose, urinalysis, and others if needed   _____

2. A. Risk factor review for coronary heart disease
   (Table _____)   _____

   B. Risk factor review for osteoporosis
   (Table _____)   _____

3. A. Early cancer detection (Checklist 3)   _____

   B. Breast exam by physician if not in past year   _____

   Pelvic examination if not in past year   _____

   Pap smear if not in past 2 years   _____

   Mammogram if not in past year   _____

4. Eye exam if not in past 2 years   _____

5. Dental exam if not in past year   _____

6. Review immunizations (p. _____)   _____

[1] Assume no other specific previous medical problems
[2] Assume no other specific previous medical problems or hysterectomy

1. A complete medical history including a discussion of any current and past medical problems.

2. A review of recent feelings and symptoms.

3. Discussion as needed of diet, nutrition, areas of stress, alcohol, tobacco and drug use.

4. A complete physical examination.

5. Laboratory tests including a complete blood count, blood chemistries including cholesterol and glucose, urine testing, and (depending on your individual situation) a chest x-ray or electrocardiogram. Chest x-ray and electrocardiogram are no longer considered a necessary part of every physical examination for every adult every year.

6. A review of your current risk factors for coronary heart disease, cancer, and in women risk factors for osteoporosis.

7. A discussion of recommendations for removal or control of any risk factors possible.

8. If any problems are present then suggestions for further studies and treatment if needed and plans for follow-up of the problem.

9. Education about any risk factors and problems found. Also, a discussion of any other questions or concerns which would help your understanding of your own health situation.

10. Hearing examinations, skin test for tuberculosis, and other tests can be planned depending on your own individual situation.

11. A complete dental examination can be discussed and planned if needed.

■ STEP TWO: BE AWARE OF BODY CHANGES

If you notice a new problem between examinations, don't wait until the next exam to notify your physician! For example, if you notice rectal bleeding, contact your physician. Suggestions for other specific problems are discussed in Chapter 5.

■ STEP THREE: IDENTIFY AND ELIMINATE RISK FACTORS

Between the more complete history and physical examinations, certain tests are very useful. These tests can continue to detect the development of new risk factors. They can also detect potential problems early for easier treatment. These can be arranged by your physician and may be done as part of your care at other visits. Some tests such as blood pressure measurement are available at many locations such as drug stores, fire stations, and shopping malls. Other tests may require a blood sample or other simple test. None of the tests are very time-consuming. It may be helpful if you keep a record of which tests you and your physician feel are useful when they are completed.

Risk factors for future disease can be identified and controlled or eliminated. Medical problems can be detected early when treatment is usually more effective and easy. Make plans now to control your future health.

■ IMMUNIZATIONS

Immunizations are available to prevent a number of diseases. Most adults received immunizations in childhood although the specific types received may not be remembered. With the help of your physician, it is useful to decide which immunizations are required to keep up to date. Some are needed only once for lifetime protection—some such as tetanus, require a booster every 10 years for protection; some, such as hepatitis B, are intended mainly for specific high risk groups. It is important to remember that many of these diseases are uncommon or rare today because of immunization. Immunization is an easy and cost-effective way to help prevent or minimize certain diseases.

Remember, each person is different. Check with your physician to see which of the immunizations are needed and safe in your own situation.

1. Influenza—Because of a higher risk of serious complications, experts recommend for all persons 65 years or older and those persons who have heart disease, many kinds of lung disease, kidney disease, diabetes mellitus, and other persons who are at higher risk of serious infection. It is recommended for health care workers and other persons who may have a higher risk of exposure to influenza.

2. Pneumococcal Pneumonia—This is commonly called the "pneumonia vaccine." Because the risk of complications of this pneumonia increases with age and up to 5 percent of serious cases may die, many experts recommend this vaccine for persons over 50 years old and for others who have heart disease, many kinds of lung disease, kidney disease, diabetes mellitus, some malignancies, some diseases in which the spleen is removed, and other diseases.

CHECKLIST 4
IMMUNIZATIONS

Immunization	Last Date Given
Influenza	_____
Pneumococcal Pneumonia	_____
Tetanus-Diphtheria	_____
Hepatitis B	_____
Rubella	_____
Measles	_____
Mumps	_____

3. Tetanus-Diphtheria—Most adults received tetanus and diphtheria immunizations as a child. A booster is needed every 10 years. If not given previously, a primary series is needed. See your physician for this.

4. Hepatitis B—This is recommended by many experts for adults who are at higher risk of exposure such as health care workers, dentists, intravenous drug users, homosexual men, dialysis patients, after exposure to Hepatitis B virus, and others. Ask your physician.

5. Rubella—Experts recommend this for adults especially women unless there is known immunization after the first birthday or a blood test shows immunity is present.

6. Measles—Experts recommend this for adults born after 1956 if not a diagnosed case of measles or if otherwise susceptible. Check with your physician.

7. Mumps—This is recommended for adults who are susceptible. Ask your physician if there is a doubt.

8. Others—Most other immunizations are for specific situations such as international travel. Check with your physician or your local health department for details about which immunizations you may need for travel, especially to developing countries. Use Checklist 4 to keep track of your immunization dates.

■ CHOOSING A PHYSICIAN

As you mature, your physician may become even more important to your well-being than ever before. Not only does your physician serve as the one who can diagnose and treat illnesses, but he or she can become a dependable friend to talk to when concerns become worries. When choosing a physician, some important factors to consider include:

1. Choose a primary physician. Some people ask friends for recommendations, check the physician's credentials, or call the local hospital for referrals. But none of these methods can be "fool-proof" in finding a person with whom you can feel comfortable to share your innermost feelings and concerns as well as provide quality medical care. Everyone needs one physician who knows the total patient. This person is able to assess your problems as a whole person and make the necessary referrals if you need further treatment or care.

2. Consider the physician's age, sex, and credentials. Know yourself when you choose a primary physician. Do you feel more comfortable with a man or woman? These questions are important to consider when making your appointment.

Ask questions with your choice of physician. Is the doctor board certified? Your local medical society can offer information. Find out if the physician has hospital privileges. Some doctors may not admit patients to certain hospitals and this might be a consideration.

3. Find a physician you can trust. Set up an appointment to talk with the physician before your examination if you feel insecure about your choice. Ask questions as to his or her methods of treatment. Does the physician relate well to people? Do you feel at ease in talking with the doctor? Are your questions answered?

4. Make sure your physician has time for you. Your physician needs to be accessible to you. When you are ill, you need to be able to see your doctor. Popularity isn't important when you are sick or in pain, but availability is. Make sure your choice of a physician is balanced with a person who is not only an excellent doctor, but one who is available to your personal needs. You can get information about emergency availability and charges. The receptionist's responses may set the tone and help you decide whether this office is for you.

■ ESPECIALLY FOR WOMEN

Women may also want to select a gynecologist, a physician who specializes in problems of women. Many women benefit greatly from the knowledge of a physician who is specially trained in this area. For example, a major decision women must make around the time of menopause is whether to take estrogen treatment. A gynecologist will be able to help make the best decision for each situation.

Gynecologists perform examinations specifically for women—a pelvic examination including examination of the vagina, cervix, uterus, Fallopian tubes, ovaries, rectum, and breasts. They deal with problems of the menstrual period, problems of fertility (difficulty in child-bearing of all kinds), avoiding pregnancy, and family planning.

Your physician can give you names of gynecologists from which to choose. Or, call your local hospital or medical society for names.

PART II

Formulating a Plan for Healthy Living

CHAPTER 4

Nutrition, Exercise, and Wellness

Good nutrition is an important preventive measure mature adults can take as they seek to play an active role in their health and well-being.

While there is certainly no guarantee that the foods you eat can prevent illness and premature death, we do know that science at least guarantees us an improved quality of life through good nutrition, as we age. By delaying the onset of illness, allowing for independent living, and reducing health care cost, good nutrition pays us back in tremendous benefits.

If you are a healthy mature adult, you can feel comfortable in knowing that the food choices you have made in years past were probably adequate for proper nutrition and disease prevention. Perhaps you have just been fortunate not to have experienced major health problems. If you are not a mature adult, but are wisely preparing for the mature years with a good nutritional foundation, you will greatly enhance your health and well-being with the proper food choices in your daily diet, thus taking preventive measures before problems begin.

Dietary habits play an important role in five of the nation's 10 leading causes of death including:

- Cancer
- Stroke

- Heart disease
- Diabetes
- Atherosclerosis

Choosing a diet consistent with the basic four food groups is vital in achieving maximum nutrition at any age, but this balanced diet is especially important as our bodies age and decline in their ability to ward off serious diseases. Even common complaints such as constipation, high blood pressure, and hemorrhoids can be prevented or controlled through proper nutrition.

■ U.S. GOVERNMENT DIETARY GUIDELINES

The 1985 Dietary Guidelines provided by the U.S. government offer some excellent suggestions to follow in optimizing your health through diet. These seven guidelines focus on actions to take to improve your diet such as:

1. Eat a variety of foods
2. Maintain desirable weight
3. Avoid too much fat, saturated fat, and cholesterol
4. Eat foods with adequate starch and fiber
5. Avoid too much sugar
6. Avoid too much sodium
7. If you drink alcoholic beverages, do so in moderation

These dietary guidelines closely parallel the recommendations made by the American Heart Association and the American Cancer Society. Please note that these guidelines are for healthy older Americans and do not apply to those who require special diets due to illness or disease. More specific individualized instruction from a registered dietitian should be sought for disease management (discussed in depth in Chapter 5).

Let's also look closely at the recommended nutrient guidelines as they apply to the life of the mature adult.

The Recommended Dietary Allowances

The Recommended Dietary Allowances (RDAs) represent the level of nutrient intake required by a healthy person to meet their nutritional needs (Table 6, 7). The RDAs are established by the National Academy of Sciences-National Research Council's Food and Nutrition Board and provide the best guide we have for determining nutrient needs.

The RDAs for adults are set up in two categories: 23 to 50 years of age and 51 plus years of age. The RDAs for those 51 plus years of age are largely estimated and based on the needs of younger adults. For years the nutrient needs of the 30-year-old have been lumped into the same category as the needs of a 65-year-old. Yet, scientists now realize that the needs of an older adult are often complicated by long-term use of medications, acute or chronic illness, and the process of aging itself. The current RDAs do not make these allowances. However, based on our present knowledge, the RDAs for older adults seem to be adequate to prevent symptoms of deficiency in most persons. In the future, the RDAs for those 51 years of age and older may need to be changed as more research sheds light on the nutrient requirements of older adults.

There are many factors that may change your nutrient needs including:

- Physical activity
- Change in body weight
- Loss of muscle
- Decline in the body's absorption of nutrients
- Chronic illness such as cancer, osteoporosis, heart disease, diabetes, or hypertension
- Surgery
- Injury
- Medications

The deficiencies of many of the nutrients including protein, some vitamins, and minerals are not uncommon in mature adults in the United States. Symptoms of these deficiencies are subtle and often accepted as part of the aging process. However, by being informed about your specific nutrient needs you can help prevent or correct these deficiencies and improve your health and well-being.

Eat a Variety of Food

Most of us recall learning the basic four food groups in elementary school. At that time, the importance of all the vitamins and minerals

TABLE 6
Recommended Daily Dietary Allowances[a]

	Age (years)	Weight (kg)	Weight (lbs)	Height (cm)	Height (in)	Protein (g)	Fat-Soluble Vitamins Vitamin A (μg R.E.)[b]	Vitamin D (μg)[c]	Vitamin E (mg α T.E.)[d]	Vitamin C (mg)
Infants	0.0–0.5	6	13	60	24	kg × 2.2	420	10	3	35
	0.5–1.0	9	20	71	28	kg × 2.0	400	10	4	35
Children	1–3	13	29	90	35	23	400	10	5	45
	4–6	20	44	112	44	30	500	10	6	45
	7–10	28	62	132	52	34	700	10	7	45
Males	11–14	45	99	157	62	45	1000	10	8	50
	15–18	66	145	176	69	56	1000	10	10	60
	19–22	70	154	177	70	56	1000	7.5	10	60
	23–50	70	154	178	70	56	1000	5	10	60
	51+	70	154	178	70	56	1000	5	10	60
Females	11–14	46	101	157	62	46	800	10	8	50
	15–18	55	120	163	64	46	800	10	8	60
	19–22	55	120	163	64	44	800	7.5	8	60
	23–50	55	120	163	64	44	800	5	8	60
	51+	55	120	163	64	44	800	5	8	60
Pregnant						+30	+200	+5	+2	+20
Lactating						+20	+400	+5	+3	+40

[a]The allowances are intended to provide for individual variations among most normal persons as they live in the United States under usual environmental stresses. Diets should be based on a variety of common foods in order to provide other nutrients for which human requirements have been less well defined.
[b]Retinol equivalents. 1 Retinol equivalent = 1μg retinol or 6 μg β carotene.
[c]As cholecalciferol, 10 μg cholecalciferol = 400 I.U. vitamin D.
[d]α-tocopherol equivalents. 1 mg d-α-tocopherol = 1 α T.E.
[e]1 N.E. (niacin equivalent) is equal to 1 mg of niacin or 60 mg of dietary tryptophan.
[f]The folacin allowances refer to dietary sources as determined by *Lactobacillus casei* assay after treatment with enzymes ("conjugases") to make polyglutamyl forms of the vitamin available to the test organism.

Water-Soluble Vitamins						Minerals					
Thiamin (mg)	Riboflavin (mg)	Niacin (mg N.E.)[e]	Vitamin B_6 (mg)	Folacin [f] (µg)	Vitamin B_{12} (µg)	Calcium (mg)	Phosphorus (mg)	Magnesium (mg)	Iron (mg)	Zinc (mg)	Iodine (µg)
0.3	0.4	6	0.3	30	0.5[g]	360	240	50	10	3	40
0.5	0.6	8	0.6	45	1.5	540	360	70	15	5	50
0.7	0.8	9	0.9	100	2.0	800	800	150	15	10	70
0.9	1.0	11	1.3	200	2.5	800	800	200	10	10	90
1.2	1.4	16	1.6	300	3.0	800	800	250	10	10	120
1.4	1.6	18	1.8	400	3.0	1200	1200	350	18	15	150
1.4	1.7	18	2.0	400	3.0	1200	1200	400	18	15	150
1.5	1.7	19	2.2	400	3.0	800	800	350	10	15	150
1.4	1.6	18	2.2	400	3.0	800	800	350	10	15	150
1.2	1.4	16	2.2	400	3.0	800	800	350	10	15	150
1.1	1.3	15	1.8	400	3.0	1200	1200	300	18	15	150
1.1	1.3	14	2.0	400	3.0	1200	1200	300	18	15	150
1.1	1.3	14	2.0	400	3.0	800	800	300	18	15	150
1.0	1.2	13	2.0	400	3.0	800	800	300	18	15	150
1.0	1.2	13	2.0	400	3.0	800	800	300	10	15	150
+0.4	+0.3	+2	+0.6	+400	+1.0	+400	+400	+150	[h]	+5	+25
+0.5	+0.5	+5	+0.5	+100	+1.0	+400	+400	+150	[h]	+10	+50

[g]The RDA for vitamin B_{12} in infants is based on average concentration of the vitamin in human milk. The allowances after weaning are based on energy intake (as recommended by the American Academy of Pediatrics) and consideration of other factors such as intestinal absorption.

[h]The increased requirement during pregnancy cannot be met by the iron content of habitual American diets nor by the existing iron stores of many women; therefore the use of 30-60 mg of supplemental iron is recommended. Iron needs during lactation are not substantially different from those of non-pregnant women, but continued supplementation of the mother for 2-3 months after parturition is advisable in order to replenish stores depleted by pregnancy.

Source: Recommended Dietary Allowances. Food and Nutrition Board, National Academy of Sciences—National Research Council, 9th rev. ed. Washington, D.C. 1980.

TABLE 7
Estimated Safe and Adequate Daily Dietary Intakes of Selected Vitamins and Minerals[a]

	Age (years)	Vitamins			Copper (mg)	Manganese (mg)	Fluoride (mg)
		Vitamin K (µg)	Biotin (µg)	Pantothenic Acid (mg)			
Infants	0–0.5	12	35	2	0.5–0.7	0.5–0.7	0.1–0.5
	0.5–1	10–20	50	3	0.7–1.0	0.7–1.0	0.2–1.0
Children	1–3	15–30	65	3	1.0–1.5	1.0–1.5	0.5–1.5
and	4–6	20–40	85	3–4	1.5–2.0	1.5–2.0	1.0–2.5
Adolescents	7–10	30–60	120	4–5	2.0–2.5	2.0–3.0	1.5–2.5
	11+	50–100	100–200	4–7	2.0–3.0	2.5–5.0	1.5–2.5
Adults		70–140	100–200	4–7	2.0–3.0	2.5–5.0	1.5–4.0

Mean Heights and Weights and Recommended Energy Intake[a]

Category	Age (years)	Weight (kg)	(lb)	Height (cm)	(in)	Energy Needs (with range) (kcal)	(MJ)
Infants	0.0–0.5	6	13	60	24	kg × 115 (95–145)	kg × .48
	0.5–1.0	9	20	71	28	kg × 105 (80–135)	kg × .44
Children	1–3	13	29	90	35	1300 (900–1800)	5.5
	4–6	20	44	112	44	1700 (1300–2300)	7.1
	7–10	28	62	132	52	2400 (1650–3300)	10.1
Males	11–14	45	99	157	62	2700 (2000–3700)	11.3
	15–18	66	145	176	69	2800 (2100–3900)	11.8
	19–22	70	154	177	70	2900 (2500–3300)	12.2
	23–50	70	154	178	70	2700 (2300–3100)	11.3
	51–75	70	154	178	70	2400 (2000–2800)	10.1
	76+	70	154	178	70	2050 (1650–2450)	8.6
Females	11–14	46	101	157	62	2200 (1500–3000)	9.2
	15–18	55	120	163	64	2100 (1200–3000)	8.8
	19–22	55	120	163	64	2100 (1700–2500)	8.8
	23–50	55	120	163	64	2000 (1600–2400)	8.4
	51–75	55	120	163	64	1800 (1400–2200)	7.6
	76+	55	120	163	64	1600 (1200–2000)	6.7
Pregnancy						+300	
Lactation						+500	

Trace Elements[b]			Electrolytes		
Chromium (mg)	Selenium (mg)	Molybdenum (mg)	Sodium (mg)	Potassium (mg)	Chloride (mg)
0.01–0.04	0.01–0.04	0.03–0.06	115–350	350–925	275–700
0.02–0.06	0.02–0.06	0.04–0.08	250–750	425–1275	400–1200
0.02–0.08	0.02–0.08	0.05–0.1	325–975	550–1650	500–1500
0.03–0.12	0.03–0.12	0.06–0.15	450–1350	775–2325	700–2100
0.05–0.2	0.05–0.2	0.1–0.3	600–1800	1000–3000	925–2775
0.05–0.2	0.05–0.2	0.15–0.5	900–2700	1525–4575	1400–4200
0.05–0.2	0.05–0.2	0.15–0.5	1100–3300	1875–5625	1700–5100

[a]Because there is less information on which to base allowances, these figures are not given in the main table of the RDA and are provided here in the form of ranges of recommended intakes.
[b]Since the toxic levels for many trace elements may be only several times usual intakes, the upper levels for the trace elements given in this table should not be habitually exceeded.

[a]The data in this table have been assembled from the observed median heights and weights of children shown in Table 6, together with desirable weights for adults given in Table 6 for the mean heights of men (70 inches) and women (64 inches) between the ages of 18 and 34 years as surveyed in the U.S. population (HEW/NCHS data).

The energy allowances for the young adults are for men and women doing light work. The allowances for the two older groups represent mean energy needs over these age spans, allowing for a 2% decrease in basal (resting) metabolic rate per decade and a reduction in activity of 200 kcal/day for men and women between 51 and 75 years, 500 kcal for men over 75 years and 400 kcal for women over 75. The customary range of daily energy output is shown for adults in parentheses, and is based on a variation in energy needs of ±400 kcal at any one age, emphasizing the wide range of energy intakes appropriate for any group of people.

Energy allowances for children through age 18 are based on median energy intakes of children of these ages followed in longitudinal growth studies. The values in parentheses are 10th and 90th percentiles of energy intakes, to indicate the range of energy consumption among children of three ages.

Source: Recommended Dietary Allowances, Food and Nutrition Board National Academy of Sciences—National Research Council, 9th rev. ed. Washington, D.C. 1980.

was not foremost in our minds as our caretakers worried about our daily diets, not us. But in order to continue the good health we enjoyed years ago, vitamins, minerals, and especially a variety of healthy foods become vital to our well-being.

A varied diet is imperative in order to receive the more than 50 essential nutrients needed to maintain health. Because no single food contains all 50 nutrients, variety is the key.

It is important to look at these nutrients so we can understand the importance of variety in the food choices we make. The 50 essential nutrients fall into six categories:

- Protein
- Carbohydrate
- Fat
- Vitamins
- Minerals
- Water

The first three nutrients—protein, carbohydrates, fats—are called the *energy nutrients*. When they are "burned" by our bodies they supply us with energy. Food energy values are expressed by calories. These three nutrients contain the following amounts of calories:

Protein	4 calories per gram
Carbohydrate	4 calories per gram
Fat	9 calories per gram

It makes sense that foods high in fat tend to be high in calories as well. For example, a teaspoon of margarine (fat) has about 35 calories, while one teaspoon of sugar (carbohydrate) has about 16 calories. This difference in calorie content can be an important factor in weight control as we tend to need fewer calories as we age. Many recent studies also show that fat control in the diet is vital in warding off diseases such as certain cancers, heart disease, and diabetes.

Protein sources include meat, poultry, fish, eggs, cheese, milk and milk products, and dried beans and peas. The role protein plays is to support the growth and maintenance of almost every cell in our body. Protein is important for the production of some hormones, maintaining the body's fluid balance and strengthening its resistance to infection. Protein can also provide energy, however, this is not its major function.

Carbohydrate sources include food containing sugar (simple carbohydrates) like candy, sodas, jelly, and jam; foods containing starch (complex carbohydrates) like bread and cereal products, potatoes, pasta, and rice; and foods containing fiber (complex carbohydrates) like bran, raw fruits and vegetables. Carbohydrates are the preferred source of energy so protein can be used for growth and the repair of body cells.

Fat sources include primarily animal fats (saturated fats) like beef and pork fat, milk fat, butter and lard; and polyunsaturated fats such as corn oil margarine, and vegetable oils. Fat provides energy, essential fatty acids and fat-soluble vitamins (A, D, E, K). Fat also makes up part of every body cell.

Vitamins are substances that are essential for normal growth, development, and the maintenance of health. They perform essential functions in the body. You are probably familiar with the water-soluble vitamins: vitamin C, thiamine (B1), riboflavin (B2), niacin (B3), and the fat-soluble vitamins: vitamins A, D, E, and K. No single food contains all the vitamins, therefore, a variety of foods are needed in the diet to assure adequacy.

Minerals are substances that are also essential for the body to perform many functions. They are required for normal growth and development and the maintenance of good health. Two familiar minerals are iron and calcium. Like vitamins, an adequate intake of minerals must come from a varied diet.

Water is essential to the body as it provides the environment in which chemical processes can take place. Water also aids in the transportation of all nutrients in the body. Water is found in the obvious sources—liquids—and also in solid food in varying amounts.

Obtaining these essential nutrients from your diet is quite simple. A balanced diet that includes foods from the following basic food groups provides the best assurance of getting all the nutrients your body needs.

Bread/Cereal Group with an Emphasis on Whole Grain Products. Four or more servings per day are recommended from this group. Examples include whole grain breads, cereals, pasta, rice, and potatoes. This group is a good source of carbohydrates, thiamine, and niacin.

Fruit/Vegetable Group with an Emphasis on Those High in Fiber. Four or more servings per day are recommended. A vitamin C source, such as orange juice, broccoli, cabbage, cantaloupe, strawberries, or citrus fruits should be included every day. A vitamin A source, such as deep orange and yellow vegetables, dark leafy green vegetables, and yellow-orange fruit should be included in the diet every other day.

Meats and Meat Substitute Group with an Emphasis on Lean Meats, Poultry, Fish and Beans and Peas. Two or more servings of this group are recommended. This group includes foods like lean red meat, poultry, fish, eggs, lowfat cheese, dried beans, and peas. These foods provide good sources of protein, iron, niacin, and thiamine.

Milk Group with an Emphasis on Lowfat or Skim Milk and Milk Products. This group includes lowfat or skim milk and milk products like yogurt. These are good sources of protein, calcium, and riboflavin, and two or more servings per day are recommended.

Fat Group with an Emphasis on the Polyunsaturated and Monounsaturated Fats. Margarine, vegetable oil, salad dressing, and mayonnaise are included in this group. These foods should be used carefully because they contribute many calories. The fat group does provide an essential fatty acid called linoleic acid.

These food groups provide the essential building blocks for our physical and mental well-being. Not only do we have to be concerned with how much protein or fat we ingest each day, there are also vitamins, minerals, trace elements, and other nutrients which are mandatory for good health. The more you can include these nutrients in your daily diet, the healthier your body will continue to be as you age.

Many mature adults are deficient in these vital nutrients because they lack knowledge or because they simply do not prepare the well-rounded meals, relying instead on convenience foods. While it may seem less costly or easier to depend on convenience foods, it is worth the extra time in preparation of fresh foods high in nutrients to enable you to maintain your good health for a longer period of time.

Protein

Protein is required for making body tissue for growth and repair. It is usually adequate in the diets of healthy older Americans (Table 8). However, long-term illness can lead to protein deficiency. This deficiency is most commonly seen in older Americans who are hospitalized for longer than 2 weeks. Surgery, chronic illness, and skin ulcerations increase the body's need for protein thus contributing to a protein deficiency. Chewing problems, digestive problems, and the inability or lack of desire to prepare food may also lead to a protein deficiency from an inadequate intake.

Symptoms of protein deficiency include weight loss, paleness, dry skin, loss of muscle, edema, fatigue, weakness, shortness of breath on exertion, and poor resistance to infection. These symptoms can also suggest other problems—cancer, medication toxicity—and should be checked out by your physician.

TABLE 8
Recommended Daily Dose (RDA) for Protein*

	Weight	Height	Calories	Protein
Female 51+	128 lbs	5′ 5″	1800	46 grams
Male 51+	154 lbs	5′ 9″	2400	56 grams

*The RDA is adequate for healthy older Americans.

Sources of Protein (Approximate)	Grams
1 ounce of meat, poultry, fish, cheese	7
1 egg	7
1 cup milk	8
1 serving bread or starch	3
½ cup beans or peas	6
½ cup of most other vegetables	2
1 serving fruit	0
1 teaspoon fat like oil or margarine	0

In the case of protein deficiency, 100 to 125 grams of protein are needed. High protein supplements—Ensure® plus high nitrogen—can be added to a regular diet to achieve this level of protein intake. Calories must be at least adequate for the body to use the protein efficiently. If you suspect a protein deficiency, consult your physician for a diagnosis and then see a registered dietitian for individualized diet instruction on a high protein diet.

Carbohydrates

Carbohydrates provide fuel or energy for the body. When adequate, they also protect dietary protein from being used for energy (Table 9). Studies have shown few problems with carbohydrate intake in healthy older Americans. However, one problem with the digestion of the milk carbohydrate, lactose, may lead to an avoidance of milk products and a diet low in calcium and vitamin D. Symptoms of this lactose intolerance include intestinal cramping, gas, and diarrhea. If you suffer

TABLE 9
Sources of Carbohydrates

Fruits	Breads and Starches
Vegetables	Sugar

from lactose intolerance and avoid milk products, be sure you get adequate calcium from other food sources or supplements.

Older Americans benefit from an increase in dietary fiber (a complex carbohydrate) since constipation is such a common complaint. Fruit, vegetable, and bran fiber should be increased, while reducing simple carbohydrates (sugar). Adding up to 10 grams of bran fiber per day to the diet has been recommended to maintain regularity and healthy bowel function.

Symptoms of carbohydrate deficiency are uncommon in the United States unless someone is on a low carbohydrate diet for weight loss or is fasting. In these cases, a condition called ketosis can occur. Without enough carbohydrates, the body turns to body fat for energy. In the process, ketones are produced (a by-product of the fat breakdown). A low carbohydrate diet resulting in ketosis is hazardous in many ways—it can cause dehydration, fatigue, irregular heartbeat from potassium losses, and blood pressure changes. A balanced, restricted calorie diet is a far better alternative for weight reduction.

There is no established RDA for carbohydrates. It has been suggested that diet include at least 500 calories from carbohydrates on a restricted calorie diet. The Committee on Dietary Allowances offers some guidelines for consideration that are in line with recommendations from other health organizations:

- Reduce intake of refined sugar since it offers no nutritional value other than a source of energy and under some conditions contributes to dental decay.
- Complex carbohydrates should be increased because they provide necessary vitamins and minerals and, in addition, are desirable for proper bowel function.

Fat

Fat is the third of the three nutrients that can provide energy. It is the most concentrated source of energy because it provides more than twice as many calories as carbohydrate or protein. Fats have a "bad reputation" because they cause weight gain, elevate your blood fats and have been linked to certain cancers. However, some fat in the diet plays an important role in being the carrier for the fat-soluble vitamins and the essential fatty acid, linoleic acid.

Current recommendations emphasize a decrease in dietary fat to reduce the risk of heart disease. In fact, dietary fat intake has declined over time in the diets of older Americans.

Symptoms of fat deficiency are rare and are usually only found in hospital patients being fed intravenously with fluids that do not contain fat. This fat deficiency is actually a deficiency in the essential fatty acid, linoleic acid. Symptoms of a linoleic acid deficiency include dry and flaky skin. This is easily reversed with the addition of fat containing linoleic acid.

There is no established RDA for fat, however, the Committee on Dietary Allowances offers some general guidelines for consideration (Table 10).

- Total fat intake should account for less than 35 percent of total calories. There should be a greater reduction of saturated fats than of unsaturated fats. However, in view of the potential hazards of a high intake of polyunsaturated fat, no more than 10 percent of the fat calories should come from polyunsaturated fat.

  More current recommendations include a cholesterol restriction. A practical interpretation of these guidelines is 30 percent of total calories should come from fat.

- 10 percent from polyunsaturated fat (most vegetable oils, and corn or safflower oil margarines)

TABLE 10
Fatty Acid Composition of Oils and Fats

| | Percent of Total Fatty Acids | | |
	Saturated	Monounsaturated	Polyunsaturated
Safflower oil	9	13	78
Sunflower oil	11	20	69
Corn oil	13	25	62
Olive oil	14	77	9
Soybean oil	15	24	61
Peanut oil	18	48	34
Sockeye salmon oil	20	55	25
Cottonseed oil	27	19	54
Lard	41	47	12
Palm oil	51	39	10
Beef tallow	52	44	4
Butterfat	66	30	4
Palm kernel oil	86	12	2
Coconut oil	92	6	2

- 10 percent from monounsaturated fat (olive oil)
- 10 percent from saturated fat (fat from animal products, shortening or hydrogenated vegetable)

The essential fatty acid and fat-soluble vitamin needs of our bodies are easily met with 2 to 4 teaspoons of fat including vegetable fats.

■ VITAMINS—WATER SOLUBLE

Folic Acid

Folate, folacin, or folic acid is one of the B complex vitamins. It functions in the body's cell growth. Folate deficiency is common in older Americans, especially in the chronically ill. Folate deficiency can also occur with long-term use of some medications and alcoholism. It may also be marginal or low in healthy persons with a low dietary intake of green leafy vegetables and breakfast cereals fortified with folacin.

Symptoms of folate deficiency can lead to one form of anemia, poor resistance to infection, fatigue, depression, confusion, forgetfulness, and poor appetite.

The RDA for folate is 400 micrograms for both men and women 51 and over. Folate is found abundantly in a variety of foods, however, a folate supplement of 400 micrograms in a multiple vitamin could be used without much risk. A supplement greater than the RDA of 400 micrograms is not recommended as it could mask the anemia that is characteristic of B12 deficiency. With any form of anemia, the cause of nutrient deficiency needs to be identified through diagnostic tests performed by your physician before any supplement is taken.

Broccoli, blackeyed peas, and orange juice are good sources of folate (Table 11).

Niacin

Niacin is needed by the body for the production of energy. A deficiency of niacin is not common among older Americans.

Symptoms of niacin deficiency include the disease pellagra which is characterized by weight loss, a rash when exposed to sun, diarrhea, irritability, and memory loss.

TABLE 11
Sources of Folate

		Micrograms
Broccoli,* frozen chopped, cooked	½ cup	153
Blackeyed peas,* frozen, cooked	⅔ cup	130
Fortified Breakfast Cereals		(variable)
Product 19	¾ cup	400
Raisin Bran, Kellogg's	¾ cup	100
Total	1 cup	400
Orange, navel	1 med.	57
Orange juice,* from frozen conc.	8 ounces	109

*Fresh broccoli, blackeyed peas, and orange juice are also good sources of folate however specific folate levels were not available.

The RDA for niacin—13 milligrams niacin equivalent—for women 51 years and older and 16 milligrams niacin equivalent for men 51 years and older. Niacin is widely available in foods (Table 12), therefore, niacin is rarely needed in a supplement. Large doses of niacin supplement can cause serious side effects, such as flushing and heart palpitations and therefore is not recommended.

Riboflavin

Riboflavin is needed by the body to produce energy. The need for riboflavin is related to calorie intake, therefore, the RDAs are lower in older adults than in younger adults. Riboflavin deficiency may

TABLE 12
Sources of Niacin

		Milligrams
All Bran, Kelloggs	⅓ cup	5
Beef, pot-roasted	3 ounces	3.6
Beef, ground chuck, cooked	3 ounces	3.4
Cornflakes, Kellogg's	1¼ cup	5
Green peas, cooked	⅔ cup	2.3
Halibut, Atlantic fresh	3 ounces	7.0
Peach, fresh	1 medium	0.9
Peanuts, w/o skin roasted	1 ounce	5.6
Potato, white baked	1 medium	1.7
Product 19	¾ cup	20

occur in older Americans with a low dietary intake. Those that do not drink milk may have a diet low in riboflavin (Table 13). Nondietary causes of riboflavin deficiency can occur in those with malabsorption, excessive use of laxatives, alcoholism, and liver disease.

Symptoms of a riboflavin deficiency include sore or burning tongue, cracks at the corners of the mouth—stomatitis—and rough, scaly skin.

The RDA for riboflavin is 1.2 milligrams in females 51 years and older and 1.4 milligrams in males 51 years and older. In a varied diet including milk products, riboflavin deficiency is not common. There is no known benefits to riboflavin supplements in large doses.

Thiamine

Thiamine is needed by the body for the production of energy. The body's need for thiamine is related to calorie intake (Table 14). Therefore the RDA for those 51 and older is lower than the RDA for younger adults. Thiamine deficiency is not a common deficiency in older Americans. However, when it occurs, the major cause is usually alcohol abuse. Thiamine deficiency has also been reported in those with cancer of the stomach and in patients on dialysis.

Symptoms of thiamine deficiency include mental confusion, poor appetite, and muscle weakness.

The RDA for thiamine is 1.0 milligrams for women 51 years and older and 1.2 milligrams for men 51 years and older. There is no evidence that large doses of thiamine provide any health benefit except in the treatment of a diagnosed deficiency.

TABLE 13
Sources of Riboflavin

		Milligrams
Beef, ground chuck cooked	3 ounces	.17
Bread, enriched	1 slice	.08
Cheese, cheddar	1 ounce	.11
Cheese, part-skim mozzarella	1 ounce	.09
Collard greens, fresh cooked	½ cup	.20
Cream of wheat, regular cooked	¾ cup	.10
Egg	1 large	.14
Milk, skim	1 cup	.34
Raisin Bran, Kellogg's	¾ cup	.4
Yogurt, lowfat	8 ounces	.49

TABLE 14
Sources of Thiamine

		Milligrams
Asparagus, cooked	⅔ cup	.16
Bread, whole wheat	1 slice	.11
Cream of wheat, cooked	¾ cup	.1
Collard greens, cooked	½ cup	.14
English muffin	1	.22
Green peas, cooked	⅔ cup	.2
Milk, skim	1 cup	.09
Oatmeal, regular cooked	¾ cup	.19
Orange juice, fresh	8 ounces	.22
Pineapple, canned in juice	1 cup	.24
Pork loin chop, cooked	3 ounces	1.01
Tomato, fresh	1 large	.12
Turnip greens, cooked	½ cup	.14

Vitamin B12

Vitamin B12 is needed by the body for the production of red blood cells and for a healthy nervous system. Overt vitamin B12 deficiency from a low dietary intake rarely occurs in mature adults because the vitamin is widely available in meats and milk products (Table 15). However, in a strict vegetarian diet (no meat, poultry, fish, eggs, or dairy products), there is an increased possibility of a vitamin B12 deficiency. Nondietary causes probably account for the vitamin B12 deficiency that exists in older Americans, occurring in up to 10 percent of those over 65. Nondietary causes such as small bowel disease, drug-nutrient interactions, alcoholism, and gastrectomy can lead to overt symptoms of vitamin B12 deficiency.

TABLE 15
Sources of Vitamin B12

		Micrograms
Chicken, without skin, roasted	3 ounces	.3
Egg	1 large	.66
Milk, skim	1 cup	.93
Tuna, white canned in water	3 ounces	1.2
Turkey, without skin, roasted	3 ounces	.3

Symptoms of a B12 deficiency include anemia, weakness, gastric upset, glossitis—a smooth, red, sore tongue—forgetfulness, irritability, tingling of the hands and feet.

The RDA for vitamin B12 is 3 micrograms. In a regular diet, B12 is readily found and deficiency is no problem. The strict vegetarian may consider supplementing the diet with 1 microgram of vitamin B12 orally, daily. This amount of vitamin B12 is often contained in a one-a-day multiple vitamin. If the vitamin B12 deficiency is diagnosed by your physician to be of nondietary cause, inadequate absorption, treatment will involve periodic B12 injections because oral supplements will not correct the deficiency.

Vitamin C

Vitamin C protects us against infection and aids in wound healing. Severe vitamin C deficiencies with symptoms are rare in the United States. However, the blood levels of ascorbic acid (vitamin C) have been found to decline with age in both men and women. This is thought to be caused by a reduced dietary intake of vitamin C, but aging may also contribute to this decline.

Symptoms of a vitamin C deficiency include loss of energy, bruising easily, gingivitis and bleeding gums.

The RDA for vitamin C is 60 milligrams. This amount of vitamin C is easy to obtain through the diet by including a few good sources daily (Table 16). A supplement of 60 milligrams of vitamin C, in a multiple vitamin preparation, can be taken if food sources of vitamin C are unavailable. In a physician-diagnosed vitamin C deficiency, larger levels of vitamin C may be given. Large doses of vitamin C taken without a deficiency are relatively nontoxic but can have some unfavorable side effects such as increased kidney stone formation, diarrhea, interference with the effects of some drugs.

TABLE 16
Sources of Vitamin C

		Milligrams
Broccoli	1 stalk	90
Orange juice	½ cup	50
Strawberries	10 large	60
Tomato	1 medium	35
Turnip greens	½ cup	70

■ VITAMINS—FAT-SOLUBLE

Vitamin A

Vitamin A is needed by the body to provide resistance to infections, to prevent night blindness, and to maintain the health of our mucosal membranes. Overt vitamin A deficiency is rare in older Americans. Symptoms of this deficiency are seldom seen in the United States because vitamin A is easily obtained from the diet (Table 17).

Symptoms of a vitamin A deficiency include poor night vision, a skin condition called dermatitis, and poor resistance to infection.

The RDA for vitamin A is 800 R.E. (retinol equivalents) for women 51+ years and 1000 R.E. for men 51+ years. There are two forms of vitamin A, one found in animal sources like fish liver oil, and beta carotene found in certain fruits and vegetables. Since vitamin A is fat-soluble, it can be stored in body fat and the liver and lead to toxicity symptoms such as headache, nausea, and blurred vision. This can be extremely dangerous, therefore, retinol (vitamin A from animal sources) supplements are not recommended. Beta carotene, the form of vitamin A found in fruits and vegetables, does not seem to cause any serious side effects except skin yellowing. However, large doses of beta carotene supplements are not recommended since it is so widely available in fruits and vegetables.

Prior to the 1980 RDAs, vitamin A was expressed in international units (ius). The most recent RDAs express vitamin A as retinol equivalents. Since most references providing the vitamin A content of food still use international units, the following information is in

TABLE 17
Sources of Vitamin A

		iu's
Apricots, canned in juice	3	1421
Cantaloupe, raw	1 cup	5158
Carrots, raw	1 large	1100
Collard greens, fresh cooked	½ cup	5400
Mustard greens, fresh cooked	½ cup	5800
Peaches, canned in juice	½ cup	475
Peaches, raw	1 medium	465
Spinach, fresh cooked	½ cup	7300
Sweet potato, baked	1 small	8100

international units. To give you a point of reference, the U.S. RDA is still 5000 ius. This is considered to be the highest level of vitamin A needed by all adults.

Vitamin D

Vitamin D is needed by the body to increase the amount of calcium available for bone formation. The dietary intake of vitamin D, in older Americans, has been found to be low. Infrequent sunlight exposure and the body's declining ability to activate vitamin D are also good reasons for a marginal vitamin D status of older Americans. The major risk in a vitamin D deficiency for older Americans is osteomalacia or adult rickets. Adequate vitamin D is important in assuring bone health.

Symptoms of vitamin D deficiency include spontaneous fractures, muscle weakness, bone pain, and accelerated loss of height.

The RDA for vitamin D is 400 ius. This can be obtained through dietary sources or from sunlight exposure, a minimum of 15 minutes twice a week (Table 18). A vitamin D supplement of no more than 400 ius, contained in a multiple vitamin preparation, is all right also. Supplemental doses of vitamin D in the form of calciferol in amounts greater than 1000 ius per day may be hazardous because this may mobilize calcium from the bones. Doses of vitamin D taken at this level and greater should only be taken under the supervision of your physician for the treatment of a low blood calcium.

Vitamin E

Vitamin E is important to the body for the maintenance of cell membranes. Vitamin E and its antioxidant effect may slow age-related changes of the body. Currently, however, there is no evidence for increasing the RDA for vitamin E with age. In healthy adults, vitamin E deficiency seldom occurs. However, older adults with intestinal disorders of malabsorption may be deficient in vitamin E.

A major symptom of vitamin E deficiency is vitamin E induced anemia.

TABLE 18
Sources of Vitamin D

		ius
Milk, fortified with vitamin D	1 cup	100
Salmon, Atlantic	3 ounces	560

The RDA for vitamin E is 8 tocopherol equivalents (1 milligram of d-alpha-tocopherol = 1 alpha-tocopherol equivalent) for women 51 years and older and 10 tocopherol equivalents in men 51 years and older. Vitamin E is readily available in vegetable oil, therefore, there is no need to supplement the diet except with a physician diagnosed vitamin E deficiency, common in malabsorption syndromes (Table 19). Vitamin E toxicity symptoms, nausea and diarrhea, can occur with supplements of 300 to 600 milligrams of vitamin E daily.

■ MINERALS

Calcium

Calcium is needed by the body for bone and teeth formation and for a healthy nervous system. Calcium is probably the nutrient most deficient in the diet of older Americans. In addition, the body's absorption of calcium also decreases with aging, particularly in women after menopause. Various medications that increase the urinary excretion of calcium, also contribute to a calcium deficiency in older Americans.

Symptoms of calcium deficiency include osteoporosis, a gradual bone loss, which can lead to spontaneous bone fractures so common among older Americans.

The current RDA for calcium is 800 milligrams for both men and women over 51 years of age. Because of new information on the calcium needs of older Americans, it has been suggested that the RDA be increased to 1000 milligrams for men and 1200 milligrams for women 51+ years of age. If this level of calcium is not consumed in a calcium-rich diet (Table 20), then a supplement of 1.5 to 2 grams (equivalent to 1500 to 2000 milligrams) calcium carbonate (40% calcium) is recommended for those at risk for osteoporosis. This level

TABLE 19
Sources of Vitamin E

		Milligrams of alpha-Tocopherol
Corn oil	1 tablespoon	1.9
Olive oil	1 tablespoon	1.6
Safflower oil	1 tablespoon	4.6
Soybean oil	1 tablespoon	1.5
Sunflower	1 tablespoon	6.1

TABLE 20
Sources of Calcium

		Milligrams
Cheese, cheddar	1 ounce	204
Cheese, part-skim mozzarella	1 ounce	183
Collard greens, cooked	½ cup	152
Milk, skim	1 cup	302
Salmon, fresh	3 ounces	258
Sardines, Pacific, canned	3 ounces	260
Yogurt, lowfat	1 cup	325

of calcium carbonate contains 600 to 800 milligrams of calcium. For mature adults with osteoporosis, therapeutic supplementation of calcium, vitamin D, sodium fluoride, and estrogen (for women) may be administered by your physician.

Iron

Iron is needed by the body's red blood cells, the hemoglobin portion, to carry oxygen to the rest of the body cells. There is little evidence that the diets of mature adults are deficient in iron (Table 21). Iron deficiency in mature adults is usually due to internal bleeding of some kind and should be checked by your physician immediately.

TABLE 21
Sources of Iron

		Milligrams
Beef, pot-roasted, lean	3 ounces	4.1
Bread, fortified	1 slice	.9
Chicken, without skin roasted	3 ounces	1.1
Cold cereals, fortified		
40% Bran Flakes	¾ cup	8.1
Product 19	¾ cup	18
Total	1 cup	18
Cream of wheat, regular cooked	¾ cup	7.5
Egg	1 large	1
Flounder, baked	3 ounces	1.2
Kidney beans, cooked	½ cup	3
Pork loin chop, lean	3 ounces	3.75
Raisins, seedless	⅓ cup	1
Turkey, without skin, roasted	3 ounces	1.5

Symptoms of iron deficiency include fatigue, paleness, and iron deficiency anemia.

The RDA for iron is 10 milligrams for men and women 51+ years. The RDA for men remains the same as younger adults, but the RDA for women is lower due to the cessation of menstruation. Iron supplements for mature adults are not routinely recommended as they mask nondietary causes of iron-deficiency anemia.

Fluoride

Fluoride is needed by the body for bone and tooth enamel formation. Some studies even indicate that fluoride may provide some protection against periodontal disease and osteoporosis. These reports remain to be confirmed. It has not been determined if the fluoride requirements for mature adults are greater than the current RDA which is the same as for younger adults.

Symptoms of fluoride deficiency include decay of the teeth and possibly periodontal disease and osteoporosis.

The RDA for fluoride is 1.5 to 4.0 milligrams for adults. No specific RDA has been established for those 51+ years of age. Even low doses of fluoride supplements cannot be recommended until further investigation. Doses of fluoride should only be used under physician supervision in the treatment of osteoporosis. Food sources of fluoride are listed in Table 22.

Potassium

Potassium is needed by the body to maintain healthy nerves and muscles. Potassium deficiency may be common in older adults, caused by

TABLE 22
Sources of Fluoride

		Milligrams
Fluoridated water		Varies—contact your local water department
Seafood		
Cod, fresh	3 ounces	.6
Mackerel, canned	3 ounces	1.0
Mackerel, fresh	3 ounces	2.3
Salmon, canned	3 ounces	.7–3.4
Vegetables grown in soil high in fluoride		(varies with location)

a diet low in potassium sources like fruits, vegetables, and milk. Medications can also cause a potassium deficiency. Diuretics like thiazide and furosemide can cause excessive loss of potassium in the urine. Poor diabetic control or the symptoms of prolonged vomiting and diarrhea can also produce a potassium deficiency.

Symptoms of potassium deficiency include weakness, poor appetite, nausea and vomiting, and confusion.

The recommended range of potassium intake is 1875 to 5625 milligrams. This need may be greater in conditions or with medications that cause an excessive potassium loss. No toxicity level is known for excessive dietary potassium. Toxicity symptoms of confusion, labored breathing, and a weakened heart can be brought on by an intravenous solution of too much potassium or the failure of the kidneys to regulate blood potassium as in kidney disease. Food sources of potassium are listed in Table 23.

Zinc

Zinc is vital to the body's resistance to infection and for tissue repair. Research studies offer conflicting data on whether mature adults are zinc deficient or whether blood levels of zinc decline with age. Many illnesses are associated with a zinc deficiency such as some cancers, kidney disease, long-term infection, trauma, and cirrhosis of the liver. Medications can also cause a zinc deficiency.

Symptoms of zinc deficiency include poor appetite, poor resistance to infection, night blindness, a decline in taste sensitivity, and skin inflammation.

The RDA for zinc is 15 milligrams for both men and women 51+ years of age. Routine zinc supplementation is not recommended

TABLE 23
Sources of Potassium

		Milligrams
Banana	1 medium	451
Figs, dried	5	665
Orange, navel	1 medium	250
Orange juice, fresh	8 ounces	496
Potato, baked	1 medium	503
Raisins, seedless	⅓ cup	375
Tomato, fresh	1 small	244
Tomato juice	8 ounces	598

TABLE 24
Sources of Zinc

		Milligrams
Beans and peas	½ cup	1.5
Eggs	2	1.0
Peanut butter	2 tbsp	1.0
Poultry, dark meat	3 ounces	2.4
Red meat	3 ounces	3.5
Skim milk	1 cup	.9
Tuna fish	3 ounces	.8

for healthy older Americans. If signs of a zinc deficiency are present, see your physician to verify that it is caused by diet alone and not a disease process. Food sources of zinc are listed in Table 24.

■ MAINTAIN A DESIRABLE WEIGHT

As we grow older, we find that winning the battle of the bulge is more and more difficult. As we age, our body functions tend to slow down and consequently our activity is on a decline. Both factors lower the calories we need to maintain a desirable weight. Calorie needs are also related to body composition which gradually changes with age. You have heard it said that everything "shifts South" as we get older. The firm, more active body tissue—muscle—slowly gives way to the soft, inactive tissue—fat. Consequently, our energy or calorie needs decline. The National Academy of Sciences (1980) recommended calorie levels for older adults to maintain desired weight (Table 25).

Table 25 is only approximate. If you feel you have a tendency toward easy weight gain, stay at the lower end of the range. If you

TABLE 25
Recommended Calorie Levels

	Age (years)	Weight (lbs)	Height (in)	Energy Needs (calories)
Men	51–75	154	71	2000–2800
	76 plus	151	71	1650–2450
Women	51–75	121	65	1400–2200
	76 plus	121	65	1200–2000

continue to be very active—walking, swimming, biking—then consume a level of calories near the high end of the range. Calorie needs in a healthy individual depend on age, sex, height, weight, and activity level. Since activity level is the only factor we can alter, increase your activity. If you aren't currently active, consult your physician before you start a strenuous work-out. When you increase your activity you not only increase your expenditure of calories (Table 26) which helps maintain your desired weight, but you also increase the blood flow throughout your body. This is quite invigorating and gives you a feeling of *well-being*. As an added bonus, some exercises such as walking, also increase the deposition of calcium in the bones which slows the development of osteoporosis.

Throughout this discussion, you may be asking yourself, "What is my desired weight?" One method to determine this is to use the 1983 Metropolitan Height and Weight Table (Table 27). You may also use the following formula:

Women: Allow 100 pounds for the first 5 feet of height, add 6 lbs for each inch over 5 feet.

Men: Allow 110 pounds for the first 5 feet of height, add 5 lbs for each inch over 5 feet.

TABLE 26
Calories Burned for Physical Activities

Type of Activity	Calories Burned per Hour (depending on weight of person)
Bicycling	300–400
Bowling	260
Calisthenics	280–350
Dancing	450–700
Gardening	350
Golf	210–300
Grocery shopping	200–300
Housework	180–240
Mowing the yard	200–350
Ping pong	360
Running	800–1,000
Sleeping	70
Stationary Biking	400–500
Swimming	350–700
Tennis	400–500
Volleyball	200
Walking	100–330

TABLE 27
1983 Metropolitan Height and Weight Table

Men

Height Feet	Inches	Small Frame	Medium Frame	Large Frame
5	2	128–134	131–141	138–150
5	3	130–136	133–143	140–153
5	4	132–138	135–145	142–156
5	5	134–140	137–148	144–160
5	6	136–142	139–151	146–164
5	7	138–145	142–154	149–168
5	8	140–148	145–157	152–172
5	9	142–151	148–160	155–176
5	10	144–154	151–163	158–180
5	11	146–157	154–166	161–184
6	0	149–160	157–170	164–188
6	1	152–164	160–174	168–192
6	2	155–168	164–178	172–197
6	3	158–172	167–182	176–202
6	4	162–176	171–187	181–207

Women

Height Feet	Inches	Small Frame	Medium Frame	Large Frame
4	10	102–111	109–121	118–131
4	11	103–113	111–123	120–134
5	0	104–115	113–126	122–137
5	1	106–118	115–129	125–140
5	2	108–121	118–132	128–143
5	3	111–124	121–135	131–147
5	4	114–127	124–138	134–151
5	5	117–130	127–141	137–155
5	6	120–133	130–144	140–159
5	7	123–136	133–147	143–163
5	8	126–139	136–150	146–167
5	9	129–142	139–153	149–170
5	10	132–145	142–156	152–173
5	11	135–148	145–159	155–176
6	0	138–151	148–162	158–179

Weights at ages 25–59 based on lowest mortality. Weight in pounds according to frame (in indoor clothing weighing 3 lbs. for women, 5 lbs. for men, shoes with 1″ heels).

Source: 1979 Build Study, Society of Actuaries and Association of Life Insurance Medical Directors of America, 1980. Reprinted with permission from Metropolitan Life Insurance Company, New York, New York.

With this method, your desirable weight could fall in a range 10 percent below or 20 percent above this weight, depending on your frame size.

Either method can give you an approximate desirable weight, however, the best weight for you is the weight at which you look and feel your best.

In trying to achieve and maintain your desirable weight, your diet plays a vital role. As mentioned earlier, as you grow older your calorie needs decline. However, you still must obtain all of the 50 or more nutrients to optimize your health. In other words, your calories must count. There is little room for those empty calories of foods high in sugar, fat, or for an excess of alcoholic beverages. The basic food groups discussed earlier present you a general plan for getting all those essential nutrients. Your energy nutrients must also be in a proper ratio so that your total calorie intake is not excessive and contributing to overweight. The following ratio is recommended for older adults in order to stay at an ideal weight:

Protein	At least 15 percent of your total calorie intake
Carbohydrate	50 percent or more of your total calorie intake with an emphasis on complex carbohydrates (whole grain products, beans, peas, fruits, and vegetables)
Fat	Less than 30 percent of your total calorie intake with an emphasis on unsaturated fat (margarines made of corn or safflower oil, liquid vegetable oils like corn oil, safflower oil, sunflower oil, soybean oil, and olive oil)

Since your calorie needs must decline with age but your vitamin/mineral needs remain at least that of young adults, you have an important task in trying to maintain your desirable weight while getting good nutrition. A rather new concept, *nutrient density*, may help you manage this balance. Foods loaded with vitamins and minerals having fewer calories are considered nutrient dense and good choices. Often the lower fat version is a more nutrient dense selection. For example, skim milk has about 80 calories per cup. Whole milk, with a similar vitamin/mineral content, has about 160 calories. The more nutrient dense choice is skim milk. This idea can also influence comparisons of different foods. For example, for a snack you could choose either a 12-ounce carbonated beverage or, for the same calories, you could have an open face grilled cheese sandwich made with lowfat cheese. The open-face grilled cheese sandwich is more nutrient dense.

■ AVOID TOO MUCH FAT, SATURATED FAT, AND CHOLESTEROL

Did you know that this year more than one million Americans will die as a result of heart disease? More than 63 million Americans suffer from one or more forms of heart and blood vessel disease. Furthermore, the American diet, high in fat and calories remains a major factor in the development of heart disease. The risk factors for heart disease including elevated blood cholesterol and triglycerides and obesity are also known to be closely linked to the type and amount of fat in the diet. A diet high in fat has also been linked to an increased risk of certain forms of cancer.

Most Americans consume a diet extremely high in fat. The typical American diet contains more than 40 percent of the calories from fat. Since fats supply over twice as many calories per gram as carbohydrate or protein, it can quickly contribute to weight gain.

- 1 gram of fat = 9 calories
- 1 gram of carbohydrate = 4 calories
- 1 gram of protein = 4 calories

While the American Heart Association recommends that Americans reduce their intake of all fats to no more than 30 percent of total calories, most people greatly exceed that figure (Table 28). Many researchers point to this high fat intake as causing a number of our chronic diseases. Think of the last time you indulged in a 10 ounce t-bone steak, potato with sour cream, broccoli with cheese sauce, and a piece of chocolate cake. This meal provides 50 percent of its calories from fat, and most of it saturated.

Watch fast foods, for example:

- Fried chicken contains 55 percent fat
- A fast food quarter-pound hamburger contains 55 percent fat
- A fish fillet doubles its calories when bathed in batter and fried in oil.

The following definitions will guide you in your attempt to reduce fat, saturated fat, and cholesterol in your diet.

Saturated fat is the fat found primarily in animal products. It is also present in foods such as whole milk, cream, butter, and cheese made from whole milk. A few vegetable fats are also highly saturated,

TABLE 28
Fat Content of Selected Foods
(By Percentage of Calories from Fat)

Foods less than 30% fat
Angel food cake
Bread
Chicken, roasted, light meat
without skin
Cod fillets, broiled
Cottage cheese, 1% fat
Crab, cooked meat
Crackers, saltines
Dried beans and peas cooked
without fat
Fruits, all—with exceptions
listed
Halibut fillets, broiled
Ice milk, vanilla
Lentils
Milk, 1% fat
Pasta
Popcorn, plain
Pretzels
Rice
Sherbet, orange
Shrimp, steamed, shelled
Skim milk
Tuna, white (albacore) canned
in water
Turkey, roasted, light meat
without skin
Yogurt, plain, low-fat
Yogurt, fruit flavor, low-fat
Yogurt, frozen
Vegetables, all—with exceptions
listed
Wheat germ

Foods 30% to 40% fat
Beef, rump—lean only
Brownie, from mix
Cottage cheese, creamed (4% fat)
Flounder, fried
Flank steak
Granola
Ice milk, chocolate
Milk, 2% fat
Shrimp, fried
Turkey, roasted, dark meat
without skin

Foods 40% to 50% fat
Chicken, roasted, dark meat
without skin
Chicken, roasted, light meat with
skin
Cookies, chocolate chip
Crackers, butter type
Cupcake with icing
Ice cream, vanilla
Milk, whole
Pork loin, lean, roasted
Salmon, canned
Tuna, white (albacore) canned in
oil
Yogurt, whole milk

Foods 50% or more fat
Avocado
Bacon
Beef rump roast, lean and fat
Bologna
Butter
Cheeses, hard such as cheddar,
swiss
Chicken, roasted, dark meat with
skin
Coconut
Coffee creamer, with coconut or
palm oil, dry powder
Cream cheese
Cream, half and half
Cream, table or light
Doughnut, cake-type
Doughnut, raised
Egg
Frankfurters
Ground beef
Ham
Margarine
Peanuts, roasted
Peanut butter
Pork loin, lean and fat
Potato chips
Salami
Sausage, pork
Sour cream
Vegetable oil
Whipped cream

such as coconut oil, palm oil (often found in nondairy cream substitutes, commercially prepared cookies, some frozen desserts) and cocoa butter (the fat in chocolate). Saturated fats tend to harden at room temperature. Vegetable oils, unsaturated by nature, can become more saturated by a process called hydrogenation. All saturated fats tend to raise blood cholesterol levels.

Dietary cholesterol is a fatlike substance found in foods from animal sources—whole milk products, meat, fish, poultry, and egg yolks (Table 29). In excessive amounts, dietary cholesterol can elevate blood level of cholesterol.

To reduce fat, saturated fat, and cholesterol, follow the suggested recommendations:

1. Buy lean meat and trim visible fat. Drain and discard the fat cooked out of the meat.
2. Fish, poultry without skin, and veal are lower in fat so consume more frequently than beef, pork, or leg of lamb.
3. Use food preparation techniques that do not require additional fat—broil, steam, bake, roast, grill, or use a small amount of fat to saute or stir-fry. Use a rack to allow fat to drain off. Baste meat, poultry, or fish with wine, broth, or lemon juice to prevent dryness. Cooking spray (corn oil) can be used to grease pans without adding a lot of fat calories.
4. Limit your consumption of organ meats like liver because of their high cholesterol content.
5. Limit your consumption of eggs to two a week (1 egg = 280 mg cholesterol). Use a commercial egg substitute or egg whites instead.
6. Avoid all highly saturated fats like butter, cream, hydrogenated margarine, shortening, coconut, and palm oil and foods made from these fats. *Read the product's ingredient list!*
7. Use skim milk or 1 percent milk instead of whole milk.

Eat Foods with Adequate Starch and Fiber

To further improve your diet, increase your intake of foods containing starch and fiber: potatoes, pasta, and whole grain bread and cereal products. These foods have an advantage over foods high in fat. You may recall that carbohydrates provide $\frac{1}{2}$ the calories of fat (1 gram of carbohydrate equals 4 calories, 1 gram of fat equals 9 calories). Starch and fiber, both complex carbohydrates, also provide the bonus of essential

TABLE 29
Cholesterol Content of Selected Foods

Food	Amount	Milligrams
Dairy		
Butter	1 tsp	11
Margarine	1 tsp	0
Skim milk	1 cup	5
1%	1 cup	10
2%	1 cup	18
Whole milk	1 cup	34
Sherbet	½ cup	7
Ice cream	½ cup	30
Cream	1 Tbsp	20
Half and half	1 Tbsp	6
American cheese	1 ounce	16
Cheddar cheese	1 ounce	30
Mozzarella, part skim	1 ounce	15
Swiss cheese	1 ounce	26
Cottage cheese, 1% fat	1 cup	10
Poultry		
Chicken, dark (no skin)	3 ounces	81
Chicken, white (no skin)	3 ounces	72
Turkey, dark (no skin)	3 ounces	87
Turkey, white (no skin)	3 ounces	66
Red meat		
Bacon	1 slice	5
Beef, lean	3 ounces	78
Frankfurter	1.6 ounces	45
Ham (boiled)	3 ounces	75
Pork (lean)	3 ounces	75
Veal (lean)	3 ounces	84
Seafood/fish		
Crab	3 ounces	85
Flounder	3 ounces	70
Haddock	3 ounces	40
Lobster	3 ounces	70
Oysters	3 ounces	42
Shrimp	3 ounces	128
Tuna	3 ounces	55
Miscellaneous		
Cereal		0
Egg noodles	1 cup	50
Egg whites		0
Egg yolk	1 large	272
Fruits		0
Nuts		0
Vegetables		0

vitamins and minerals. Fiber gives foods volume and bulk and will satisfy a hearty appetite with fewer calories. For example, which do you think would make you feel fuller: 1 ½ cups air-popped popcorn or 1 pat of margarine? They both contain about 45 calories. Popcorn is a complex carbohydrate while margarine is pure fat.

Complex carbohydrates are found in beans, peas, fresh fruits, vegetables, and whole grain bread and cereal products. These foods are much better for you than foods high in simple carbohydrates such as sugar. Simple carbohydrate foods provide calories but little else in the way of nutrients or fiber, with the exception of fruit juices.

Including more complex carbohydrates in your diet has definite health advantages. Fiber tends to reduce constipation, diverticulosis, and may lower your risk of colon cancer. It may also lower blood cholesterol levels. Unfortunately, Americans only consume an average of 10 to 15 grams of dietary fiber daily. The National Cancer Institute recommends 20 to 35 grams of dietary fiber per day. To increase the fiber in your diet, make a goal to double your intake (Table 30). Here are some ways to increase the amount of fiber in your diet:

1. Buy whole grain bread, not white bread.
2. Buy fresh fruits and vegetables. Eat more raw fruits and vegetables. If you cook your vegetables, steam or stir-fry them until

TABLE 30
Fiber Content of Selected Foods

	Amount	Grams
Breads		
Bran muffin	1 average	3
Pumpernickel	1 slice	2
Rye	1 slice	2
White	1 slice	1
Whole wheat	1 slice	2
Cereals		
Cream of wheat, instant	1 ounce	1
Cheerios	1 ounce	2
Fiber One	1 ounce	12
Grits, uncooked	¼ cup	4.8
All Bran	1 ounce	9
All Bran with extra fiber	1 ounce	14
Bran flakes	1 ounce	4
Corn flakes	1 ounce	1

TABLE 30 (Continued)

	Amount	Grams
100% Bran	1 ounce	10
Oat bran	1 ounce	4
Oats, uncooked, rolled	½ cup	4.5
Raisin Bran	1 ounce	3.5–4
Grape Nuts	1 ounce	2
Dried fruits		
Dried dates, medium	2½	1.5
Dried fig, medium	1½	4.5
Dried prunes, medium	3	4
Raisins	2 Tbsp	1.2
Fruits		
Apple (with skin)	1 medium	3
Banana	1 medium	1.5
Cantaloupe, cubes	1 cup	2
Cherries, raw	12	1
Grapefruit	½ medium	2.5
Grapes	15	.5
Orange	1 medium	2
Peach, raw	1 medium	1.5
Pear, raw	1 medium	2.8
Plum, raw	2 small	1.5
Strawberries, raw	1¼ cup	6.5
Tangerine	1 medium	2
Watermelon, cubes	1¼ cup	1.75
Vegetables		
Beans, green	½ cup	1.5
Beets, cooked	½ cup	1.6
Broccoli, cooked	½ cup	1.1
Cabbage, cooked	½ cup	1.5
Carrots, cooked	½ cup	1.4
Carrots, raw	1 medium	3.7
Cauliflower, cooked	½ cup	1.2
Cauliflower, raw	1 cup	1.8
Corn, kernel	½ cup	3.2
Kale, cooked	½ cup	2
Kidney beans, cooked	½ cup	7
Lettuce	1 cup	1
Peas, cooked	½ cup	4
Potato, baked	1 with skin	3.5
Spinach, raw	½ cup	2
Summer squash	½ cup	2.2

crisp, not soft and mushy. (Steaming also retains their vitamin and mineral content.)

3. Consume fruits and vegetables with edible skins left on them for added fiber.
4. Select brown rice over polished white rice or instant rice.
5. Enjoy the vast selection of legumes in your diet. (However, avoid seasoning them with animal fat.)
6. Select a breakfast cereal high in fiber (3 or more grams per serving) to start your day off.

Fiber Food Diary

You can get an accurate account of how much fiber you take in each day by recording the foods you eat and the fiber content. (See Checklist 5.) Use the listing given on fiber content in foods and keep a total of a week's food intake in this diary. Do you meet the amount of fiber required by your body each day or the 20 to 35 grams as recommended by the National Cancer Institute?

Avoid Too Much Sugar

Syrup, jam, jelly, candy, cookies, cakes, pies, soft drinks, ice cream, and sweetened cereals all have at least one ingredient in common—sugar. Foods high in sugar are considered simple carbohydrates. These foods often tend to be in concentrated forms of calories and therefore not included in weight-loss diets. Consider the sugar content of these foods (Tables 31, 32).

In addition, some sweetened cereals are more than 60 percent sugar by weight. Frequently, the ingredients list on the label of the product will provide a clue to its sugar content. (Remember, ingredients are listed in order of contents by weight. The first listing is the most predominant ingredient.)

Sugar may be in the form of glucose, maltose, dextrose, lactose, sucrose, xylitol, sorbitol, fructose, corn syrup, or corn sweeteners. Be a discerning consumer and read the ingredients list on products.

To avoid sugar, follow these guidelines:

1. Read the ingredients list of the food product to determine sugar content. Select an alternate product without added sugar. For example, select a water-packed can of fruit over one packed in syrup.

CHECKLIST 5
FIBER FOOD DIARY

Day	Food Item	Serving Size	Fiber Amount
Monday	_____	_____	_____
	_____	_____	_____
	_____	_____	_____
	_____	_____	_____
	_____	_____	_____
	_____	_____	_____
Total for Day:			_____
Tuesday	_____	_____	_____
	_____	_____	_____
	_____	_____	_____
	_____	_____	_____
	_____	_____	_____
	_____	_____	_____
Total for Day:			_____
Wednesday	_____	_____	_____
	_____	_____	_____
	_____	_____	_____
	_____	_____	_____
	_____	_____	_____
	_____	_____	_____
Total for Day:			_____
Thursday	_____	_____	_____
	_____	_____	_____
	_____	_____	_____
	_____	_____	_____
	_____	_____	_____
Total for Day:			_____

CHECKLIST 5 (Continued)

Day	Food Item	Serving Size	Fiber Amount
Friday	_____	_____	_____
	_____	_____	_____
	_____	_____	_____
	_____	_____	_____
	_____	_____	_____
Total for Day:			_____
Saturday	_____	_____	_____
	_____	_____	_____
	_____	_____	_____
	_____	_____	_____
	_____	_____	_____
Total for Day:			_____
Sunday	_____	_____	_____
	_____	_____	_____
	_____	_____	_____
	_____	_____	_____
	_____	_____	_____
Total for Day:			_____

TABLE 31
Sugar Content of Selected Foods

Food	Amount	Sugar Content
Cola	12 ounces	9 teaspoons
Jelly	1 tablespoon	6 teaspoons
Iced cupcake	1	6 teaspoons
Flavored gelatin	½ cup	4½ teaspoons

TABLE 32
Sugar Content of Cereals

Cereal*	Amount	Grams
All Bran, extra fiber	1 ounce	0.0
Bran Chex	1 ounce	5.0
Buc Wheats	1 ounce	9.0
Cornflakes	1 ounce	2.0
Crispex	1 ounce	3.0
Cracklin Bran	1 ounce	8.0
Frosted Mini Wheats	1 ounce	6.0
Fruit Loops	1 ounce	13.0
Golden Grahams	1 ounce	10.0
Mueslix	1 ounce	6.5
Nutrific Oatmeal	1 ounce	8.0
Puffed Wheat	1 cup (14 grams)	0.0
Puffed Rice	1 cup (14 grams)	0.0
Rice Krispies	1 ounce	3.0
Shredded Wheat	1 ounce	0.0
Sugar Frosted Flakes	1 ounce	11
Sugar Smacks	1 ounce	16
Total	1 ounce	3.0
Total Raisin Bran	1 ounce	9.0

*1 ounce of cereal equals 28 grams.

2. Use products sweetened with non-nutritive sweeteners (calorie free) like aspartame (Equal) or saccharine (Sweet-n-Low).

3. Select a sugar-free or low sugar cereal.

Here is a sample ingredients list from a cereal. How many sugars can you identify? We've italicized the sugars—there are five.

RAISIN BRAN

Ingredients: Wheat bran with other parts of wheat, raisins, *sugar*, tricalcium and dicalcium phosphate (provides calcium), *brown sugar syrup*, *cereal malt syrup*, salt, *honey*, *corn syrup*, zinc, and iron (mineral nutrients), vitamin E (dl-alpha-tocopherol acetate), trisodium phosphate, a B vitamin (niacinamide), vitamin C (sodium ascorbate), a B vitamin (calcium pantothenate), vitamin A (palmitate), vitamin B6 (pyridoxine hydrochloride), vitamin B2 (riboflavin), vitamin B1 (thiamine mononitrate), a B vitamin (folic acid), vitamin B12 and vitamin D, freshness preserved with BHT.

Avoid Too Much Sodium

Did you know the average American consumes about 2 to 4 teaspoons of salt per day (4400 to 8800 mg sodium)? The body actually needs only about ½ to 1½ teaspoons of salt per day (1100 to 3300 mg sodium). Reducing the amount of salt in your diet can help some people avoid high blood pressure. People with high blood pressure are more likely to develop heart disease and stroke. Although the words "salt" and "sodium" are often used interchangeably, they are not the same. Ordinary table salt is only 40 percent sodium. The other 60 percent is another mineral, chloride. It is the sodium part of salt that is necessary to maintain water balance in body tissues. However, too much sodium can increase fluid retention and elevate blood pressure in people who are sodium sensitive.

Many foods naturally contain sodium including animal products like meat, fish, poultry, milk, and eggs (Table 33). Vegetable products are naturally low in sodium. Most of the sodium in our diets, however, comes from commercially processed foods such as cured meats like bacon and ham; luncheon meats; sausage; frozen breaded meats, fish, and seafood; and canned meats and fish. Condiments like catsup, mustard, and steak sauce are also high in sodium. Fast foods such as a hamburger, french fries, and prepare-at-home fast foods like broccoli with cheese sauce are very high in sodium. Start reading the ingredients list on the label of the package to determine the sodium content.

Words that have soda, sodium, or "Na" associated with them indicate sodium as a part of a preservative or flavoring agent. Some examples are monosodium glutamate, baking soda, sodium nitrate, sodium propionate, and sodium benzoate.

Since 1985, the U.S. Food and Drug Administration has required nutrient labels on food packages to list the sodium content. Terms such as "low sodium" and "sodium free" were also standardized to help the conscientious consumer:

Sodium free	Less than 5 mg sodium/serving
Very low sodium	35 mg or less sodium/serving
Low sodium	140 mg or less sodium/serving
Reduced sodium	Sodium reduced 75% compared to the product it is replacing
Unsalted, no salt added	Sodium has not been used in processing

TABLE 33
Sodium Content of Selected Foods

Food	Amount	Milligrams
American Cheese	1 ounce	400
Bacon	2 slices	200
Baking powder	1 tsp.	339
Baking soda	1 tsp.	821
Beans, green	½ cup	230
Beef broth	1 cube	1150
Beef, lean	3 ounces cooked	55
Bread	1 slice	150
Biscuit	1 (2″ diameter)	220
Buttermilk	1 cup	330
Cereal, dry, flake	⅔ cup	200
Cheeseburger, fast food	¼ lb.	1200
Chicken noodle soup	1 cup	1100
Cornbread	1 small square	260
Cheese, cheddar	1 ounce	200
Choc. shake	1 average	300
Cottage cheese	4 ounces	450
Frankfurter	1½ ounces	500
Garlic powder	1 tsp.	1
Garlic salt	1 tsp.	1850
Ham	3 ounces	1000
Ketchup	1 tbsp.	156
Lite salt	¼ tsp.	250
Luncheon meat	1 slice	575
Mayonnaise	1 tbsp.	80
Meat tenderizer	1 tsp.	1750
MSG, flavor enhancer	¾ tsp.	50
Mozzarella, part-skim	1 ounce	132
Mustard	1 tsp.	65
Oatmeal, instant	¾ cup	240
Oatmeal, regular	¾ cup	1
Olives, green	3	720
Onion powder	1 tsp.	1
Onion salt	1 tsp.	1620
Peas, green canned	1 cup	493
Peas, green frozen	1 cup	150
Potato, boiled	1 cup	7
Potato, instant	1 cup	475
Potato chips	1 ounce	300
Peanut butter	1 tbsp.	100
Sauerkraut	⅔ cup	740
Sausage, pork	2 links	380
Salt	¼ tsp.	500
Soy sauce	1 tbsp.	1030
Tomato juice	½ cup	210

Remember, sodium is measured in grams and milligrams. A gram is a unit of weight. There are about 28 grams in one ounce. One gram equals 1000 milligrams. The American Heart Association recommends no more than 1000 to 3000 milligrams (mgs) sodium per day.

To avoid high sodium intake:

1. Avoid excessive amounts of sodium by using fresh, frozen vegetables (no salt added), or canned vegetables (no salt added).

2. Use fresh meats, fish, chicken instead of canned or processed meat like luncheon meat (ham, bologna, bacon, sausage).

3. Avoid the use of convenience box mixes (macaroni and cheese, scalloped potatoes, dressing mixes) and frozen convenience foods (TV dinners, vegetables in white or cheese sauces, frozen potato products, even low calorie frozen dinners are high in sodium and should be used with caution for those on sodium restriction).

4. Read the ingredients list of food products to determine sodium content (ingredients are listed in order of contents by weight). Some packages even provide the number of milligrams of sodium per serving.

5. Use herbs, commercial salt-free seasonings, salt substitute, lemon juice, or vinegar to flavor foods.

6. Avoid fast foods. If you find you must eat at a fast food restaurant, eat from the salad bar.

If You Drink Alcoholic Beverages, Do So in Moderation

Excessive alcohol consumption for most, provides a lot of extra calories and very little in the way of nutrients. In fact, alcohol interferes in the absorption of some nutrients contained in food. A few beers every day can quickly equal a "beer belly." For others, alcoholic beverages alter the appetite and becomes a substitute for a good diet. This deprives the body of all the essential nutrients needed to maintain good health. Long-term malnutrition and impaired resistance to infection can result in hospitalization and leads to major medical bills. Alcohol can also increase your risk for throat cancer and cirrhosis of the liver.

Finally, anyone on medication, prescription or over-the-counter, should use caution in drinking any alcoholic beverage. Alcohol may interfere with the effectiveness of the drug or even multiply its effect.

■ SUGGESTIONS FOR REDUCING ALCOHOL CONSUMPTION

Allow yourself just one mixed drink, light beer, or one glass of wine or champagne, then switch to lemon-flavored seltzer or mineral water over ice, or a diet soda.

Drink your favorite mixed drink minus the alcohol. You might not miss it!

HEALTHY DIET QUIZ

Rate the health of your diet with the following questionnaire. Answer each question by marking yes or no.

	Yes	No
1. I mainly eat meat and potatoes.		
2. I know my desirable weight.		
3. I use skim or lowfat milk.		
4. My breakfast cereal is a whole grain cereal.		
5. I drink my tea and coffee without any sugar.		
6. I salt my food before tasting it.		
7. I drink mainly on the weekends and then I lose count.		
8. I eat at least two servings of vegetables every day		
9. I eat chicken, fish and potatoes fried.		
10. I eat white bread rather than whole wheat.		
11. I drink regular soft drinks.		
12. I use only foods prepared naturally instead of convenience foods (t.v. dinners, vegetables in sauces).		
13. I abstain from all alcohol.		
14. I eat fish and/or chicken frequently for supper.		
15. I am overweight by at least 10% of the desirable weight (see Table 27).		
16. I use a corn oil or safflower oil margarine.		
17. I like my vegetables cooked until they are soft.		
18. I eat a dessert containing sugar every day.		
19. I season my food with a variety of herbs instead of salt.		
20. I have at least two alcoholic beverages every day.		
21. I eat canned soups regularly.		
22. I have a citrus fruit or juice just about every day.		
23. I eat eggs and bacon or sausage almost every morning for breakfast.		
24. I eat dried beans or peas several times a week as a meat substitute.		

	Yes	No
25. I often skip a meal and eat something sweet (cookies, cake, frozen yogurt, or ice cream) instead.	——	——
26. I include luncheon meats, ham, hot dogs, sausage, or canned meats in my diet regularly.	——	——
27. I enjoy the produce (fresh fruits and vegetables) in season.	——	——
28. I avoid milk and dairy products.	——	——
29. I have red meat just about every meal.	——	——
30. I eat 2 or more pieces of raw fruit every day.	——	——

Score

Score your questionnaire by giving yourself one point for each correct answer.

1. no	11. no	21. no
2. yes	12. yes	22. yes
3. yes	13. yes	23. no
4. yes	14. yes	24. yes
5. yes	15. no	25. no
6. no	16. yes	26. no
7. no	17. no	27. yes
8. yes	18. no	28. no
9. no	19. yes	29. no
10. no	20. no	30. yes

Score

27–30	Congratulations! You have a HEALTHY diet.
23–26	You are almost there with just a few changes.
19–22	Typical diet—could use improvement.
15–18	Come on. Shape up! You're ailing!
15 or less	Help! Reread Chapter 4 now!

CHAPTER 5

Nutrition
and Disease

E very day, researchers are finding out more about the role of foods
and nutrients in preventing major diseases. While the studies
are not complete, there is enough speculation to make us aware of
the impact good nutrition and a healthy lifestyle have on our overall
well-being.

Our diet greatly effects the way we feel. Too much of one type
of food may cause lethargy, too little of some foods may bring on
nutritional deficiencies resulting in symptoms of weakness or nausea.
Not only is a balanced diet important for good health, diet plays a key
role in assisting the person who is diagnosed with illness or diseases.

The foods you eat for prevention of disease and during times of
illness or disease can assist you in coping with treatment, tolerating
medications, and boosting your immune system to the point where it
can continue to fight off other illnesses.

Let's look at some common diseases that may affect you or someone you know and the role a nutritionally sound diet plays in prevention and treatment.

■ CANCER

It is estimated that 50 percent of all types of cancer in women and 30
percent in men are associated with environmental factors—radiation,
ultraviolet rays from the sun, chemicals, smoking, diet. Diet has been
estimated to cause 35 percent of all cancers. As discussed in Chapter 3,
diet change and not smoking can provide us with the best prevention

for cancer or at least delay its occurrence. Certain foods and the vitamins and minerals contained in these foods may provide prevention against cancer.

■ REDUCING YOUR RISK OF CANCER THROUGH NUTRITION

Alcohol. Excessive amounts of alcoholic beverages have been linked to a number of forms of cancer—cancer of the mouth, throat, esophagus, and liver. Smoking and drinking together increase the risk of mouth and esophageal cancer even more. There may be a link between alcohol consumption and breast cancer, however, more research is needed in this area. Moderation seems to be the key—limit your alcoholic beverages, including beer, to 1 to 2 drinks per day.

Calcium. Preliminary studies suggest that calcium plays a protective role against cancer of the colon. In a long-term study, milk drinkers had less than 1/2 the incidence of colon cancer than non-milk drinkers. Possibly, the calcium in milk neutralizes potential cancer-causing substances. Calcium is found in abundance in lowfat milk and milk products like cheese, yogurt, and ice cream. If you are lactose intolerant and cannot consume dairy products, consult your physician for a calcium supplement. Refer to Table 34 for more information about calcium supplements.

Cruciferous Vegetables. Broccoli, brussels sprouts, cauliflower, cabbage, kohlrabi, rutabagas, and turnips are members of the cruciferous family of vegetables. They are thought to contain chemicals that activate an enzyme in the body's intestines that breaks down cancer-causing agents, thus preventing the development of cancer.

Fat. Fat accounts for 40 to 45 percent of the total calories in the typical American diet. A 12-year study by the American Cancer Society found a link between a high fat diet and an increased risk of 5 of the 6 most common forms of cancer—breast, cervix, colon, rectum, and prostate. Other studies also suggest that excessive dietary fat will increase your risk of cancer.

To reduce your risk of cancer, cut back on the amount of fat in your diet, both saturated and polyunsaturated. Limit your fat calories to less than 30 percent of your total calorie intake.

TABLE 34
Some Calcium Supplements

Name	Type of Calcium	Actual Amount of Calcium
Tums tablets	Calcium carbonate 500 mg/tablet	200 mg/tablet
Tums E-X tablets	Calcium carbonate 750 mg/tablet	300 mg/tablet
Digel tablets	Calcium carbonate 280 mg/tablet	112 mg/tablet
Alkamints tablets	Calcium carbonate 850 mg/tablet	340 mg/tablet
Biocal calcium supplement tablets	Calcium carbonate 1250 mg/tablet	500 mg/tablet
Biocal calcium supplement chewables	Calcium carbonate 625 mg/tablet	250 mg/tablet
Calcium carbonate tablets, generic	Calcium carbonate 500 mg/tablet	200 mg/tablet
Calcium carbonate oral suspension	Calcium carbonate 1250 mg/tsp.	500 mg/tsp.
Cal-Sup tablets	Calcium carbonate 750 mg/tablet	300 mg/tablet
Dorcal children's liquid supplement	Glubionate calcium 1800 mg/tsp.	115 mg/tsp.
Neo-Glucagon syrup	Glubionate calcium 1800 mg/tsp.	115 mg/tsp.
Os-Cal 500 tablets	Oyster shell, 1250 mg	500 mg/tablet
Calcium gluconate tablets, generic	Calcium gluconate 500 mg	45 mg/tablet
Calcium lactate tablets, generic	Calcium lactate 650 mg	84.5 mg/tablet
Titralac tablets	Calcium carbonate 420 mg/tablet	168 mg/tablet

For example, if you consume 1800 calories you can determine your fat calories as follows:

1800 calories × 30 percent fat calories = 540 calories from fat per day

To determine the number of grams of fat allowed per day divide by 9 calories per gram of fat:

540 fat calories / 9 calories per gram of fat = 60 grams of fat per day.

This same information can also be useful in making sense out of food product labels. For example, a food product has 180 calories per serving and 10 grams of fat. To determine the percentage of calories from fat in this food product, do the following calculation:

10 grams of fat $\times$ 9 calories per gram of fat = 90 fat calories

90 fat calories / 180 calories per serving = 50 percent calories from fat.

This food product is obviously high in fat and way beyond your goal of 30 percent calories from fat. Be careful not to be misled by labels that read "90% fat-free." These labels may be referring to weight and not calories, so look for the nutrition information and calculate percentage of calories from fat. Often these products are high, 50 percent or more calories from fat. More and more food manufacturers are providing this kind of nutrition information for the consumer. Take advantage of this information in your attempt to keep fat calories to 30 percent or less of your total calories.

A practical approach to reducing your dietary fat, both saturated and polyunsaturated, includes consuming skim milk and skim milk dairy products, very lean meat, fish, or skinless poultry, plenty of fruits and vegetables, and whole grain products. Limit your use of margarine, butter, shortening, oil, bacon—all fats. Also avoid the hidden fat in chips and other snack foods, rich desserts, salad dressings, sauces, and gravies. Finally, switch your food preparation techniques from frying to broiling, baking, roasting, and poaching.

Fiber

People who eat food that is high in dietary fiber have a lower incidence of colon cancer, the second most common form of cancer in the United States. Most Americans consume less than 15 grams of dietary fiber per day while the National Cancer Institute recommends 20 to 35 grams of dietary fiber per day. To increase your fiber intake include more foods high in fiber such as fresh fruits and vegetables, whole grain bread and cereal products, whole grain pastas, brown rice, dried beans, nuts and seeds. Obtain different types of fiber by including a wide variety of foods *without* reliance on fiber supplements.

Food Preparation/Processing

Food preparation techniques such as charcoal grilling can produce cancer-causing agents in food. A safer method of grilling includes wrapping the food in foil or in a pan and then on the grill. Any method that prevents the flames and smoke from coming in contact with the food is safer than putting food directly on the grill.

Food processing techniques such as salt curing, pickling, and smoking have also been shown to increase the incidence of stomach cancer in areas where these foods are consumed in large quantities. This may explain why stomach cancer is so common among the Japanese. Nitrite cured meats have also been implicated as a cancer-causing substance, however, this risk is lowered when the diet includes fruits and vegetables rich in vitamin C.

Obesity

An American Cancer Society study showed that people who were more than 40 percent overweight had an increased risk of cancer of the colon, breast, prostate, gall bladder, ovary, and uterus. Other populations studies have also shown this association. To lose weight and keep it off, attempt to lose it slowly—1 to 2 pounds per week. The best method is to cut calories by reducing the amount of fat in your diet and EXERCISE!

Vitamin A

Beta-carotene, a form of vitamin A, occurs naturally in food and works in the body by ensuring the health and growth of the cells of the mucous membranes. People who consume a diet low in beta-carotene have a higher incidence of cancer than those who eat a diet rich in beta-carotene. There is an association between reduced risk of lung cancer and the consumption of foods rich in beta-carotene. To increase your intake of foods abundant in beta-carotene eat more of the following: apricots, broccoli, cantaloupe, spinach, sweet potatoes. *Warning*: Beta-carotene from food sources is virtually nontoxic, however, do not take vitamin A supplements in other forms as they can be toxic and cause liver damage when taken in excess.

Vitamin C

Vitamin C, like beta-carotene, may prevent the formation of cancer-causing chemicals like nitrosamines. (Nitrosamines are produced when preservatives like nitrites, used in processed meats, are broken down in the body.) Despite the existing evidence linking vitamin C to cancer protection, it should be pursued further in research. Vitamin

C sources include broccoli, brussels sprouts, cabbage, cantaloupe, citrus and citrus juices, collard greens, green pepper, kale, mustard greens, tomatoes, and strawberries.

Vitamin E

Vitamin E, like vitamin C, with the mineral selenium may control cell damage caused by substances called "free radicals" and may reduce the risk for cancer development. These results have only been observed in animal studies and therefore require further investigation. *Warning:* Selenium is toxic in large doses and produces severe consequences. *Do not* use supplements. Consume only the food sources of selenium as well as of vitamin E. Vitamin E sources include wheat germ, whole grains and cereals, vegetable oil and products made with vegetable oil. Selenium food sources include grain products grown in selenium rich soil and seafood.

Summary of Dietary Recommendations of the American Cancer Society

1. Limit the total fat in the diet.
2. Eat more fruits and vegetables especially those rich in vitamins A and C. Eat vegetables from the cabbage family (cruciferous family).
3. Increase the amount of fiber in your diet.
4. Drink alcohol in moderation.
5. Maintain desirable body weight and exercise.
6. Consume salt-pickled, cured, smoked, and nitrite-cured foods in moderation.

The statistics are encouraging that almost 50 percent of those diagnosed with cancer will be alive at least 5 years after diagnosis. If a person has cancer and must undergo treatment for the disease including therapies such as chemotherapy, radiation, immunotherapy, and surgery, it is proven that the well-nourished person fares best. Treatments are often more effective in the well-nourished person, because higher levels of chemotherapy or radiation can be used. A well-nourished person also recovers from surgery faster and with fewer complications. Unfortunately, a person with cancer may find it hard to eat well, and weight loss and poor resistance to infection can result.

■ WEIGHT LOSS WITH CANCER

Weight loss is a major nutritional problem in the cancer patient. Often the treatment, chemotherapy or radiation, can reduce appetite and cause symptoms like altered taste sensations that hinder eating. The cancer itself or even surgery can also cause weight loss. Finally, the depression that is associated with a diagnosis of cancer, can reduce appetite and cause weight loss. When weight is lost, the body compensates for the lack of nutrients and energy by breaking down its own muscle and internal organs to meet the body's needs. Therefore, weight loss and muscle wasting must be prevented in the cancer patient.

If the person with cancer has a poor appetite and cannot eat much food at one time, it is vital that what little food is eaten be very nutritious—high in calories and protein. The main goal through any cancer therapy should be to keep body weight stable or even to gain weight. The dietary goal of the cancer patient should be to start out eating an adequate diet including the following list of foods, and then add to this diet from the suggestions given next.

1. Have at least 2 servings of milk or milk products daily such as ice cream, pudding, flavored yogurt, or cheese.
2. Eat at least 2 to 3 servings of fruit or fruit juice every day. Include one serving of a fruit with vitamin C like orange juice.
3. Include at least 2 servings of vegetables per day. One should be a good vitamin A source, yellow or green leafy vegetables.
4. Eat at least 2 servings of meat, poultry, or fish daily.
5. Include four or more servings of bread and cereal.
6. Include nutritious snacks like cheese, peanut butter, nuts, and desserts as desired to boost calorie and protein intake.

■ WAYS TO BOOST YOUR CALORIE AND PROTEIN INTAKE

- Take a walk or drink a beer or glass of wine prior to mealtime to stimulate your appetite.
- Eat small meals more frequently to increase your intake. Keep foods out to snack on throughout the day and include a bedtime snack.

- Save your favorite foods for periods when your appetite is poorest.
- Protein foods often taste bitter to people with cancer, so try eating protein foods cold or at room temperature in the form of cheese, tuna, or chicken salad, ham or egg salad, luncheon meat, deviled eggs, milkshakes, puddings, custards, or commercial nutritional supplements.
- Add powdered milk to milkshakes, puddings, custards, and casseroles to increase the protein and calorie content of the food.
- Fortify your whole milk by adding 1 cup of dry milk to 1 quart of fluid milk. This addition doubles the protein content of the milk.
- If meat is tolerated, marinate it in a variety of spices to enhance flavor. Use sugar and salt (if allowed by physician) as desired. Or try a marinade of fruit juice or wine.
- Use extra butter or margarine to add calories to foods. Sour cream, cream cheese, mayonnaise and whipped cream are also high in fat and calories so use them liberally.
- Foods high in carbohydrates are often readily consumed and can add calories to the diet. They include popsicles, jelly and jam, honey, flavored gelatin, marshmallows and other candies.

If you experience a bitter or metallic taste in your mouth, suck on hard candy or drink fruit juice or ginger ale to cut it.

■ USING NUTRITIONAL SUPPLEMENTS

Nutritional supplements can also be used to boost the calorie and protein intake of the diet. The list in Table 35 includes those supplements that are free of the milk carbohydrate lactose which may cause diarrhea and gas in those that are lactose intolerant.

Those supplements which contain milk are listed in Table 35.

In choosing a nutritional supplement, you need to consider individual taste and economics. If the person undergoing cancer treatments has experienced any gas or diarrhea, then the lactose-free supplements should be chosen until the symptoms have disappeared. Most of these supplements can be found in your local pharmacy. However, if the store does not stock the supplement you desire, then request that the pharmacist get it for you. Most pharmacists will accommodate this request. Instant Breakfast (found in most grocery stores) is by far the least expensive supplement, however, it is mixed

TABLE 35
Nutritional Supplement

Product	Company
Ensure (a liquid)	Ross
Ensure Plus (a liquid)	Ross
Enrich (a liquid)	Ross
Resource (a mix)	Sandoz
Sustacal (a liquid)	Mead Johnson
Sustacal High Calorie (a liquid)	Mead Johnson
Supplements containing milk	
Meritene (a liquid or a mix)	Sandoz
Sustacal (mix with milk)	Mead Johnson
Sustagen (mix with milk)	Mead Johnson
Instant Breakfast (mix with milk)	Carnation

with milk and therefore contains milk carbohydrate, lactose. All supplements may be more appealing if they are mixed with ice cream or fruit to make a milkshake.

Constipation

Besides weight loss and poor appetite, the person with cancer may suffer from constipation. It may be caused by the cancer itself or the therapies used to combat the disease. The rationale for the dietary suggestions is to increase the fiber and fluid content of the diet to relieve constipation. As mentioned earlier, wheat bran fiber seems to be the most effective fiber in relieving constipation. Wheat bran adds bulk to the stool and increases the rate of movement of the stool through the bowel. To relieve constipation:

1. Increase fiber intake by consuming raw vegetables and fruits, bread and cereals containing wheat bran and dried fruits. If chewing is a problem then grate, shred and blenderize fruit or vegetables and add to juices, gelatin or cereal.
2. Include at least 8 to 10 glasses of fluid per day.
3. Relax after meals.
4. Use warm or hot liquids to stimulate peristalsis (bowel activity).
5. Exercise to your ability and as allowed by your physician.

If constipation continues to be a problem consult your physician about a stool softener.

Diarrhea

Diarrhea can be caused by the cancer itself, the therapy used to combat the disease or malnutrition. Cancer can cause diarrhea, depending on the type and location of the cancer. Radiation and chemotherapy are also known to interfere with the normal function of the intestinal tract. These therapies hinder the regeneration of the intestinal tract, which results in diarrhea. Malnutrition can also change the intestinal tract lining and cause diarrhea as a consequence.

To minimize diarrhea follow these dietary suggestions:

1. Avoid the gas producing vegetables such as cabbage, cauliflower, dried beans and peas.
2. Use cooked fruits and vegetables rather than raw or fresh.
3. Decrease your intake of the fiber containing foods such as nuts, seeds, produce with tough skins, whole grain bread and cereals.
4. To replace fluids and potassium losses from diarrhea, use fruit juices and nectars, popsicles, Gatorade®, fruit ices, and bananas.

Nausea and Vomiting

Nausea and vomiting can be caused by the cancer or by the therapy used in treating the cancer. The nausea from chemotherapy should subside within 24 to 48 hours after the treatment. With radiation therapy, nausea usually occurs 2 hours after each treatment and subsides shortly thereafter. The feelings of fullness and nausea may be decreased by limiting the volume of food in the stomach at one time. Nausea can also be minimized by avoiding strong odors from food as it is prepared.

To minimize nausea and vomiting follow these recommendations:

1. Eat small, frequent meals or snacks.
2. Try dry foods (i.e., toast, crackers).
3. Use cool or warm liquids to get you through periods of nausea (i.e., ginger ale, clear soups, gelatin, popsicles, or fruit slushes).
4. Use liquids between mealtimes rather than at mealtimes.
5. If you rest after a meal, elevate your head or rest in a sitting position.
6. Avoid preparing foods having a strong odor.

7. Eat in a room other than where the food is prepared to avoid the odor.

8. Eat slowly and chew foods well.

9. Avoid fried or greasy foods while nauseated.

10. Avoid exercising after eating.

11. Change to a clear liquid diet if nausea persists; report it to your physician.

Chewing/Swallowing Difficulties

Radiation and chemotherapy can create problems that interfere with chewing and swallowing. Radiation of the head and neck can decrease the amount of saliva secreted resulting in xerostomia (dry mouth). Radiation and chemotherapy can also lead to stomatitis, mouth ulcers, and esophagitis all of which makes chewing and swallowing painful.

The rationale of these dietary suggestions is to encourage the consumption of moist, easily chewed and swallowed foods. Known food irritants should be avoided.

1. Include plenty of fluids; 1 to 2 quarts a day.

2. Moisten foods with gravies and sauces to aid in swallowing.

3. Use mints or lemon drops to stimulate saliva production.

4. Chop, grate, or blenderize foods. (Heat foods first then blenderize.)

5. Use foods which are cool or warm rather than extreme temperatures.

6. Avoid acid fruits; try apple, pear, peach and banana.

7. Use a straw for liquids of thin blenderized foods.

8. Try popsicles or frozen juices.

9. Avoid spicy, salty, or coarse foods and alcohol.

10. Soak foods in liquids for a more tender texture.

11. Tilt head back to ease swallowing.

12. Use moist foods, casseroles, macaroni and cheese, yogurt; blend if desired.

■ CORONARY HEART DISEASE (CHD)

The National Heart, Lung and Blood Institute states that 40 million Americans are at risk for CHD with cholesterol levels of 240 mg/dl or greater. It is known that blood cholesterol levels increase with age.

Blood cholesterol levels tend to rise until age 60 for men and until age 70 for women. Elevated blood cholesterol is the major risk factor for CHD. Elevated serum cholesterol levels can be reduced by limiting the saturated fat and cholesterol content of the diet. By lowering your blood cholesterol level, you dramatically reduce your risk of CHD. Other risk factors for CHD include high blood pressure, smoking, diabetes, family history of premature CHD, and obesity.

To reduce your risk of CHD, follow these summarized dietary recommendations. A healthy heart diet change is not temporary; it must be a lifestyle change if the results are to lower your risk of heart disease for a lifetime.

Practical Strategies to Lower Your Risk of Heart Disease

1. Limit your intake of fat-marbled red meats. Use lean cuts of red meats and then trim any visible fat. Eat more fish and skinless poultry. Keep portion sizes of meat or poultry to 2 to 4 ounces.

2. Limit your intake of egg yolks to 2 to 3 a week. Substitute 2 egg whites for each egg yolk in cooking and baking.

3. Substitute whole milk products with their skim milk counterparts.

4. Cook with a polyunsaturated oil (corn, safflower, or sunflower oil) and use a polyunsaturated margarine (corn or safflower oil are listed as the first ingredient in the ingredients list), instead of lard, butter, or shortening.

5. Use a monounsaturated oil like olive oil in salad dressings, pasta, and vegetable salads.

6. Use vegetable protein sources instead of meat frequently. For example, 1 cup of dried beans or peas have about as much protein as 2 to 3 ounces of cooked meat, but much less fat. Combine with rice or wheat bread to make the protein equivalent to meat protein.

7. Avoid frying foods, instead use cooking methods that do not require fat like broiling, baking, microwaving, roasting, and stewing. Stir frying is acceptable if the food is prepared in a small amount of unsaturated vegetable oil.

8. Avoid eating fatty luncheon meats, hot dogs, and sausage.

See Table 36 Lean Choice Substitutions.

TABLE 36
Lean Choice Substitutions

If you are currently using:	Try these alternatives:
Butter	Reduced calorie corn oil margarine
Cheese	Lowfat cheese
Ground beef	Ground round
	Ground sirloin
	Ground turkey
Luncheon meat	Lowfat luncheon meat
Mayonnaise	Reduced calorie mayonnaise
Oil	Vegetable oil cooking spray
Salad dressing	Oil free or reduced calorie salad dressing
Sour cream	Drained lowfat yogurt (To drain yogurt, line a strainer with paper towel or cheese cloth. Place yogurt in strainer and allow to stand for 30 minutes.)

■ HIGH BLOOD PRESSURE

Hypertension or high blood pressure is very common in those over 50 and is a contributing factor to the leading cause of death and disability, coronary heart disease. There are many predisposing factors for high blood pressure as discussed in Chapter 2.

Alcohol

There is increasing evidence of a link between excessive alcohol drinking and high blood pressure. Research has shown that for those drinking four or more drinks per day, there is a significant rise in the incidence of high blood pressure.

Other Dietary Factors

Diet influences the onset and severity of high blood pressure. Being overweight is known to elevate blood pressure. Sodium restriction may protect against the onset or delay the progression of high blood pressure. Many health organizations, including the American Heart

Association, have made recommendations for reducing sodium in the diet for the general public (1 gram of sodium per 1000 calories consumed per day).

Other dietary factors may also effect blood pressure. Minerals, such as chloride or magnesium, may also play a role in the prevention and/or management of high blood pressure. Excessive saturated fat in the diet may elevate blood pressure. Potassium, calcium, polyunsaturated fat and fiber may lower or maintain normal blood pressure. Not enough evidence exists to make more specific dietary recommendations in regard to high blood pressure.

Blood Pressure Management with Diet

1. Weight Loss—if you are overweight or obese since blood pressure increases with the increase in body weight.
2. A sodium restriction of 2 to 3 grams sodium (or 2000 to 3000 milligrams). Excessive sodium in the diet has been associated with high blood pressure in the sodium sensitive person.
3. Decrease your intake of saturated fat because persons with high blood pressure often have elevated cholesterol levels and an increased risk of heart disease. Two types of drugs often used to control blood pressure, thiazide diuretics and beta-blocking agents, may also elevate blood lipids.
4. Regular exercise.
5. Limit alcohol to 2 ounces per day. Consumption of more alcohol than this is associated with high blood pressure.
6. Caffeine is known to elevate blood pressure for the short-term, however, it has not been associated with inducing permanent high blood pressure. You may want to avoid caffeine if you will be having your blood pressure checked, otherwise moderation is the key.

Sodium Restriction

The words *salt* and *sodium* are often used interchangeably, however, they are not the same. Table salt (sodium chloride) is 40 percent sodium and 60 percent chloride. Salt largely contributes to the sodium in our diet, however, foods and drugs also contain other forms of sodium. Sodium is frequently used as a preservative in foods. (See Chapter 4, p. 107.) When possible, select the lower sodium alternative as listed in Table 37.

TABLE 37
Lower Sodium Food Alternatives

Avoid	Acceptable
Canned vegetables	Low sodium or salt-free canned vegetables, fresh vegetables, or frozen without salt
Processed meats like luncheon meat, bacon, sausage, hot dogs, corned or chipped beef, bacon, sausage, smoked fish, canned meats, potted meats, anchovies, caviar, sardines	Fresh meats are a much better alternative. If you must use a processed meat occasionally, use the lower salt or lower sodium version.
Boxed convenience foods, pizza, macaroni and cheese, potato dishes	Prepare homemade using low sodium products like low sodium tomato sauce, low sodium cheese.
Breads and cereals	Select bread without a salted top
Instant cereal	Cold cereals. Hot cereals and rice should be long cooking, not instant.
Soups, and gravies, bouillon, dehydrated soup and gravy mixes	Prepare homemade without adding salt or select the low-sodium version at your grocery store.
Snack foods like chips, pretzels, crackers, peanuts, popcorn	Select the unsalted version at your grocery store.
Frozen meals	Prepare homemade and freeze portions for later use. Frozen dinners are high in sodium.
Seasonings and condiments, meat tenderizers, garlic salt, onion salt, soy sauce, worcestershire sauce, lite salt, pickles, olives, chili sauce, steak sauce, lemon-pepper, barbecue sauce, dips and spreads	Use the salt-free herb seasonings available in your grocery store or see the chart that follows and create your own seasonings from the abundant variety of herbs and spices. Only use a salt substitute at the discretion of your physician because they are high in potassium. Catsup and mustard may be used in small amounts (1 teaspoon).

Remember that a person with high blood pressure who responds to sodium restriction should try to stay below 2 to 3 grams of sodium per day.

A Practical Approach to a Moderate Sodium Intake

1. Cut by half the amount of salt you consume. This can be achieved by using a little salt to cook with and then avoid added salt at the table (remove the salt shaker from the table).

2. Try to use more herbs, commercial salt-free seasonings, lemon juice or vinegar to flavor foods instead of salt.

3. Choose fresh or frozen vegetables or purchasing no salt added canned vegetables.

4. Use fresh meats, fish, chicken rather than canned or processed meats like luncheon meat (ham, bologna, bacon, sausage . . .).

5. Use convenience box mixes infrequently (macaroni and cheese, scalloped potatoes, dressing mixes . . .) and frozen convenience foods (TV dinners, frozen vegetables in white or cheese sauces, frozen potato products), even low-calorie frozen dinners are high in sodium.

6. Limit your visits to fast food restaurants as most fast food is higher in sodium than the same food prepared at home. If you must eat at a fast food restaurant, then have the salad bar.

■ DIABETES

The preventive effect of diet on diabetes shows great promise. A diet low in simple carbohydrate (sugar), low in fat, moderate in protein, and moderate to high in complex carbohydrate (especially fiber-containing foods like whole grain bread and cereal products, vegetables, and fresh fruits) is suggested. The Dietary Guidelines for Americans reviewed in Chapter 4 are a good place to start.

Obesity has also been strongly associated with elevated blood sugar and adult-onset diabetes. Achieving and maintaining desirable weight is imperative.

Glucose metabolism (the body's breakdown and utilization of carbohydrate) slows down with age leading to elevated blood glucose or blood sugar and diabetes. Approximately 25 percent of persons 65 years or older have elevated blood sugar or even diabetes. Diabetes is a major risk factor in atherosclerosis (hardening of the arteries), one of the major causes of illness and death in older Americans.

In the milder form of diabetes, noninsulin dependent type II diabetes, dietary treatment contributes to the optimum management of blood sugar level, blood cholesterol and triglyceride levels, and body weight. It also minimizes the need for drug therapy to manage these problems, saving money and suffering from the side affects of medication.

Goals in the dietary management of noninsulin dependent type II diabetes includes good control of blood sugar level, blood cholesterol, and triglyceride levels and the maintenance of desirable body weight.

The achievement of these goals can be measured in your physician's office during a routine check-up. Ask your physician for your lab results and weight.

For the dietary management of diabetes, the American Diabetes Association has made these recommendations:

- Consume a level of calories to achieve and maintain desirable body weight.
- Determine your desirable weight by using the Metropolitan Height/Weight Chart (Table 27).
- Carbohydrates should make up 55 percent of your total calories with an emphasis on fiber-containing foods (whole grain bread and cereal products, vegetables, and fresh fruits). Carbohydrate foods low in fiber should be avoided (desserts made with refined white flour and sugar, candy, regular soft drinks, jam and jelly, breads and cereals made with refined white flour, alcohol).
- Fiber, a complex carbohydrate, is believed to have some influence on blood sugar control in diabetes. Studies have shown improved blood sugar control with a high carbohydrate, high fiber diet. The water-soluble fibers (pectins from fruits, gums from beans and peas, and oat bran) seem to delay glucose or sugar absorption in the gastrointestinal tract allowing for a slow release of sugar to the blood. This prevents elevated blood sugar peaks and stabilizes diabetes.

  These same water-soluble fibers also reduce elevated blood cholesterol, common among diabetics. Studies have shown 15 to 30 percent reduction in blood cholesterol levels in consumers of water-soluble fibers. This is equivalent to a 30 to 60 percent reduction in the risk of heart disease.

Adequate dietary fiber, 25 to 35 grams, can easily be obtained by including a variety of foods such as cooked beans and peas, whole grain bread and cereal products, oatmeal, oat bran cereals, oat bran breads and muffins, plenty of fresh fruits and raw vegetables.

- 15 to 20 percent of the total calories should be from protein (meat, seafood, poultry, skim milk, and skim milk products like lowfat cheese, yogurt, and eggs). Protein sources should be low in saturated fat and cholesterol, as diabetics are at greater risk for heart disease.

- Total fat and cholesterol should be restricted. Total fat should be restricted and comprise less than 30 percent of total calories. Cholesterol should be restricted to less than 300 milligrams per day. Saturated fat (primarily animal fat and hydrogenated vegetable fat) should be substituted with unsaturated fats (polyunsaturated margarine or vegetable oil, and monounsaturated fat like olive oil). This recommendation may slow the development of atherosclerosis (hardening of the arteries) so common in diabetics. For suggestions in reducing saturated fat and cholesterol in the diet see recommendations in Chapter 4.

- Use saccharin or aspartame instead of sugar to prevent elevating the blood sugar dramatically.

  The American Diabetes Association recommends 1000 milligrams of sodium per 1000 calories not to exceed 3000 milligrams per day. This is especially important to the hypertensive diabetic. For suggestions in reducing sodium in the diet see Chapter 4.

- Use alcoholic beverages with caution as specific problems of hypoglycemia, obesity, poor blood sugar control, elevated blood fats can result from too much. Alcohol should be avoided if the blood triglycerides are elevated.

- Vitamins and minerals should meet the current Recommended Dietary Allowances (Chapter 4). There is no evidence that a diabetic requires additional vitamins or minerals unless a specific deficiency is identified or the diabetic is on a very low calorie diet for weight loss.

■ DIGESTIVE DISEASES

Currently, many national health care organizations such as the American Heart Association, the American Cancer Society, National Cancer

Institute recommend increasing the complex carbohydrates and fiber in your diet to lower your risk of constipation, diverticular disease, hemorrhoids. It is estimated that direct medical costs in treating these gastrointestinal diseases run Americans more than 17 billion dollars per year. Annual sales of prescription and over-the-counter medicines for digestive diseases run 1.2 billion with 450 million being spent for laxatives alone. To find a method of prevention for the painful symptoms of digestive diseases would not only save billions of dollars but also relieve many chronic sufferers. Below are some specific recommendations based on the latest in research findings.

Constipation

Chronic constipation may contribute to the development of other digestive diseases—diverticular disease and hemorrhoids. Increasing fiber in the diet has shown a consistent benefit in regulating bowel movements. The water-insoluble fibers, particularly wheat bran, have a marked laxative effect by increasing the rate of movement of a stool through the intestines. Consumption of plenty of fluids, exercise, and stress reduction can also improve your regularity.

Diverticular Disease

Research data indicates that persons consuming a diet low in fiber are more likely to develop diverticular disease. Insoluble fibers from vegetables and whole grain bread and cereal products, especially wheat, increase the stool's bulk and water content, thereby softening the stool. This tends to reduce the incidence of diverticular disease. Fiber is also helpful in the treatment of diverticular disease once it occurs.

Increasing the fiber in your diet may cause gas, abdominal cramping, and loose bowel movements. The best strategy for increasing fiber to the National Cancer Institute's recommended 20 to 35 grams per day, is to do it gradually (over 5 to 6 weeks). This slow introduction of fiber will allow the gastrointestinal tract time to adapt. Remember, moderation is the key; an excessive amount of fiber can also interfere with the gastrointestinal tract's absorption of minerals.

■ OSTEOPOROSIS

In order to delay or even prevent osteoporosis, you need to be sure to have enough calcium in your diet. See Chapter 2 for a complete discussion of the disease osteoporosis, and refer to Table 34 for calcium supplements.

Ways to Increase the Calcium in Your Diet

1. Include 3–4 servings of calcium-rich products in your diet daily. Milk, cheese, and yogurt all contain lactose which enhances calcium absorption.
2. If you are counting calories, do not exclude dairy products, but select lowfat or skim milk products.
3. Vitamin D also enhances intestinal absorption of calcium. Therefore, sun exposure, which allows the body to make vitamin D, and drinking vitamin D-fortified milk can be helpful.
4. Avoid a diet high in fat and protein as excessive fat and protein can interfere with calcium absorption in the intestines.
5. Avoid an excessive intake of soft drinks and convenience foods containing food additives as high levels of phosphorus and phosphates can result in calcium loss from the bone.
6. Other sources of calcium include salmon with bones, sardines, and green leafy vegetables like broccoli. However, the oxalate content of the green leafy vegetables, like spinach, may decrease the absorption of calcium.
7. Caffeine in coffee has also been implicated in calcium loss, so avoid excessive use.

■ RHEUMATIC DISEASE OR ARTHRITIS

Although researchers have yet to find a cure for most types of arthritis, they have realized the importance of diet in weight reduction which may alleviate some of the pain and swelling in the joints.

Overweight has a significant impact on arthritic-strickened joints of the lower body. Research has shown that weight loss relieves the severity of arthritic symptoms. Achieving desirable weight is encouraged for the arthritic.

■ HEALTHY KITCHEN CHECKLIST

Knowing that good nutrition can affect prevention and treatment of most major illnesses, you need to take a survey of your kitchen cabinets. How healthy is your kitchen? Are the foods on your grocery list in line with the Dietary Guidelines for Americans? See Checklist 6.

CHECKLIST 6
HEALTHY KITCHEN CHECK

Yes	No
Skim or 1% milk	Whole milk
Part-skim cheeses—mozzarella, ricotta	Cheeses made with whole milk
Reduced fat cheeses (<5 grams of fat per ounce)	
Lowfat cottage cheese	
Lowfat yogurt	
Fresh fruit, fruits canned in their own juices, unsweetened fruit juice, dried fruits	Sugar coated fruits and fruit fillings, canned fruits in syrup
Raw vegetables, steamed vegetables or vegetables cooked crisp	Vegetables cooked soft or cooked with meat fat
Skinless poultry, fish, very lean cuts of red meat, reduced fat luncheon meats (<5 grams of fat per ounce)	Commercial sausage, bacon, regular luncheon meat, hot dots, fat marbled red meats
Whole grain bread and cereal products, crackers with unsalted tops, unsalted popcorn	White bread, refined breakfast (low fiber), salted or flavored crackers, popcorn or nuts
Unsaturated vegetable oils, (corn, safflower, sunflower, soybean, olive), margarines made with liquid corn oil or safflower oil	Excessive amounts of saturated fat (animal fats, shortening, hydrogenated fats)
Commercial egg substitute, egg whites	Whole egg, egg yolk
Vegetable oil based salad dressings, low calorie or oil-free salad dressing	Creamy or cheesy salad dressings (sour cream cheese based dressings)
Fruit juice popsicles, sherbet, Angel food cake, homemade bran muffins, homemade oatmeal cookies for those at desired weight	Commercial baked goods (pies, cakes, cookies), ice cream, packaged cookies containing palm, coconut or hydrogenated oils

CHAPTER 6

Food
and Drug
Interactions

Medication plays an important role in the treatment and management of many physical problems. Many people are living longer and more productive lives due to medicine, however, medication can become a serious problem when it is not taken as directed. Medication reactions can often seem worse than the ailment that it is intended to treat.

Americans take almost 40 billion doses of medication each year, and older Americans take more medication than any other group. The changing health of many mature adults requiring daily medication places this age group at a higher risk for the adverse reactions of some drugs and foods. This risk of food-drug interactions is due to the age-related changes that occur in the body's use and clearance of medications. Long-term use of medications and the use of several medications at one time can greatly increase this chance of adverse food and drug reactions. Because the mature adult's kidneys and liver cannot process drugs as quickly as a younger adult, an even greater threat of adverse reactions and drug overdoses occurs.

The consequences of a food-drug reaction range from constipation to actually bringing about a full-blown vitamin or mineral deficiency. Let's look at how medications can interfere with the body's state of nutrition:

- Cause a poor or uncontrollable appetite.
- Enhance or hinder the body's absorption of vitamins and minerals and the other nutrients.
- Change the way the body uses vitamins and minerals and the other nutrients.
- Change the rate at which the body gets rid of vitamins and minerals and the other nutrients.

■ BE AWARE OF DRUG-NUTRIENT INTERACTIONS

By being aware of possible drug-nutrient interactions and food-drug interactions that can occur in your drug regimen, you can minimize the adverse effects of medications. Food can influence the absorption of your medication so it is wise to know how a medication should be taken. The state of your stomach can decrease, delay or even increase the absorption of your medication. See Tables 38, 39, 40, 41.

Another example of the interactions of your diet and your drug therapy can occur with alcohol use. Alcoholic beverages are frequently included in the diet even while on medications. There are several dramatic consequences of alcohol on the effectiveness of a medication (Table 42):

TABLE 38
Food and Drug Interactions: Poor Absorption of Nutrients

Drugs That May Cause Poor Absorption	Nutrients Poorly Absorbed
Antibiotics	
Tetracycline HCl	Calcium
Neomycin	Fat, calcium, sodium, potassium, iron and vitamin B12
Antacids	
Aluminum hydroxide	Phosphate, calcium
Anticonvulsant	
Phenytoin (Dilantin)	Calcium
Antiinflammatory Drugs	
Colchicine	Fat, nitrogen, vitamin B12
Laxatives	
Phenolphthalein	Fat, calcium, potassium
Mineral oil	Vitamin A, vitamin D, vitamin K, betacarotene

TABLE 39
Food and Drug Interactions:
Altered Use of Nutrients

Medications that may change
the way the body uses nutrients:

Hydralazine is a vitamin B-6 antagonist

Isoniazid is a vitamin B-6 antagonist

Methotrexate is a folacin antagonist

TABLE 40
Food and Drug Interactions: Rapid Loss of Nutrients

Drug	Minerals Lost
Antacids	
Aluminum Hydroxide	Phosphate
Antiinflammatory Drugs	
Aspirin	Iron
Diuretics	
Hydrochlorothiazide	Potassium, zinc, magnesium
Furosemide	Potassium, magnesium, calcium
Laxatives	
Phenolphthalein	Potassium, calcium

TABLE 41
Drug-Food Interactions

Drugs Which Are Better Absorbed on an
Empty Stomach:

Penicillin G (Oral)	Isoniazid
Cephalexin	Tetracycline
Erythromycin (Stearate)	Aspirin
Phenacetin	Theophylline

Drugs Which Are Better Absorbed with
Food or Milk:

Erthomycin (Ethylate)	Nitrofurantoin
Propranolol	Griseofulvin
Chlorothiazide	Prednisone
Indocin	Levodopa
K-Lor	K-Lyte

TABLE 42
Possible Alcohol-Drug Interactions

Drug Type	Possible Reactions
Antianginal	Dangerous drop in blood pressure
Antibacterial	Increased risk of liver toxicity
Antibiotic	Liver damage, similar to Antabuse reaction
Anticoagulant	Alters drug effect
Anticonvulsant	Deep sedation, provokes seizures, liver damage
Antidepressant	Excessive intoxication
Antidiabetic, oral	Similar to an Antabuse reaction
Antidiarrheal	Decreased brain function
Antifungal	Increased risk of liver damage
Antiglaucoma	Increased alcohol/brain effects
Antihistamine	Excessive sedation
Antihypertensive	Dangerous blood pressure drop Increased sensitivity to alcohol
Antihyperthyroid	Increased liver toxicity
Antimicrobial	Similar to an Antabuse reaction
AntiParkinson	Increased alcohol effect
Antiprotozoal	Similar to an Antabuse reaction
Antipsoriatic	Likely liver damage
Antiviral	Brain and nerve damage
Appetite suppressant	Dangerous rise in blood pressure
Cortisone	Increased ulcer risk
Diuretics	Dangerous drop in blood pressure
Hypnotic/Sedative (Barbiturates)	Fatal over sedation, excess drug effects
Immunosuppressant	Intestinal bleeding
Insulin	Increased drug effect-hypoglycemia, brain damage
Muscle relaxants	Depresses brain activity

- Increase or decrease absorption of the medication by the gastrointestinal tract.
- Interactions changing the way the body uses the medication, sometimes with side effects. (Alcohol taken with some medications can cause symptoms similar to the reaction caused by the alcohol deterrent, Antabuse. These symptoms include vomiting, rapid heart beat and chest pains.)

Before accepting a prescription from your physician, inform him of any past drug reactions you experienced, the medications you are currently using, and your medical history—current or previous conditions—such as heart disease, high blood pressure, diabetes or kidney disease.

■ HOW TO MINIMIZE FOOD AND DRUG INTERACTIONS

There are preventive measures you can take to ensure the least possible interaction between food and the drugs you must take. Some medications must be taken immediately following a meal while others must be taken on an empty stomach. If rules such as these are broken, the results can often be worse than the illness being treated. Certain medications cannot be mixed with alcohol or the end result can be deadly. Be sure to contact your physician if you have any questions concerning your medication and possible reactions, and follow the pharmacist's instructions on each prescription and over-the-counter medication you take.

Antacids

Aluminum Hydroxide (Amphojel). Take one to three hours after a meal. May cause a decreased absorption of vitamin A, phosphorus and an inactive thiamine. May cause constipation.

Aluminum Hydroxide and Magnesium Hydroxide (Maalox). Take with water between meals. May cause a decreased absorption of calcium and phosphorus with long-term use. May cause constipation.

Calcium Carbonate (Tums). Take one to three hours after a meal as an antacid. Diet Recommendations: As a calcium supplement, avoid taking with foods high in oxalates—whole grain bread and cereal products, bran. May cause nausea and constipation.

Dihydroxyaluminum Sodium Carbonate (Rolaids). Take one to three hours after a meal. May cause constipation.

Sodium Bicarbonate, Potassium Citrate (Alka-Seltzer). Dissolve in water. Diet Recommendations: High in sodium for those on a sodium restricted diet—296 milligrams of sodium in each tablet.

Antacid/Pain Reliever

Sodium Bicarbonate, Sodium Citrate, Aspirin (Alka-Seltzer). Dissolve in water. Diet Recommendations: High in sodium for those on sodium restricted diet—554 milligrams of sodium in each tablet. Do not use if allergic to aspirin, or if you have asthma or a bleeding disease.

Antibiotics

Ampicillin (Polycillin).   Take on an empty stomach, one hour before or two to three hours after a meal. Diet Recommendations: Avoid alcohol. May cause loss of appetite, nausea or diarrhea.

Cephalosporin (Ceclor, Keflex).   Take with food especially with stomach upset. Diet Recommendations: Avoid alcohol. May cause nausea, vomiting or diarrhea.

Erythromycin (E-Mycin, Erythrocin).   Take with water on empty stomach, one hour before a meal or two or three hours after a meal. May cause nausea.

Penicillins (Bicillin, Pen G Sodium).   Take with water on empty stomach, one hour before a meal or two to three hours after a meal. Diet Recommendations: Avoid acidic fruit juices at time of medication. May cause nausea, vomiting, or diarrhea.

Sulfonamides (Bactrim, Septra).   Take with water on empty stomach, one hour before a meal or two or three hours after a meal. Diet Recommendations: Drink plenty of fluids and avoid alcohol. May cause loss of appetite. May cause nausea, vomiting, or diarrhea.

Tetracycline (Tetracyn, Achromycin).   Take on empty stomach, one hour before or two hours after a meal. Diet Recommendations: Avoid antacids and dairy products such as milk, cheese, and yogurt as they decrease the body's absorption of the medication.

Antihistamines

(Periactin, Chlortrimeton, Benadryl).   Take on a full stomach to avoid stomach irritation. Diet Recommendations: Avoid alcohol. Beverages with caffeine may reduce side effect of drowsiness.

Arthritis/Anti-inflammatory Medications

Allopurinol (Zyloprim).   Take after meals with plenty of fluids. Diet Recommendations: Avoid alcohol. Drink plenty of fluids.

Ibuprofen (Motrin, Advil, Nuprin).   Take with meals or milk.

Diet Recommendations: Avoid alcohol. May cause poor appetite, nausea, vomiting, constipation, and fluid retention.

Indomethacin (Indocin).   Take with meals or milk. Diet Recommendations: Avoid alcohol. May cause poor appetite, nausea, vomiting, and headache.

Naproxen (Naprosyn).   Take with meals. Diet Recommendations: Avoid alcohol. May irritate mouth, cause constipation, weight gain.

Penicillamine (Cuprimine).   Take on empty stomach one hour before or two to three hours after a meal. Diet Recommendations: Drink plenty of fluids. May cause poor appetite, nausea, vomiting, or diarrhea.

Blood Thinning Medication or Anticoagulants

Dipyridamole (Persantine).   Take on an empty stomach with water, at least one hour before or two to three hours after a meal. May cause nausea, vomiting and gastric upset.

Warfarin (Coumadin).   Diet Recommendations: Avoid alcohol and limit caffeine. Avoid foods high in vitamin K (leafy green vegetables, liver, egg yolks, soy oil, and fish). May cause gastric upset.

Blood Pressure Medications

Captopril (Capoten).   Take on an empty stomach, one hour before or two to three hours after a meal. Diet Recommendations: Physician may prescribe low calorie, low sodium diet as appropriate. May cause dizziness. Physician should monitor blood levels of sodium and potassium.

Clonidine (Catapres).   Diet Recommendations: Avoid alcohol. Physician may prescribe low calorie, low sodium diet as appropriate. May cause drowsiness, nausea, and constipation.

Hydralazine HCl (Apresoline).   Take on full stomach at the same time every day. Diet Recommendations: Physician may prescribe low sodium diet. May cause poor appetite and gastric upset.

Propranolol HCl (Inderal).   Take on full stomach. May cause nausea, vomiting, dizziness, and constipation. Diet Recommendations: Physician may prescribe low calorie, low sodium diet as appropriate.

Resperine (Sandril).   Take with food or milk. May cause gastric upset. Diet Recommendations: Physician may prescribe low calorie, low sodium diet as appropriate. May cause nausea, vomiting, and poor appetite.

Cancer Medications

See Chapter 5 on the management of symptoms during chemotherapy.

Bleomycin Sulfate (Blenoxane). Given as an injection or intravenously (iv). May cause stomatitis, nausea, vomiting, and poor appetite.

Cyclophosphamide (Cytoxan). Given as an injection, through an iv, or by mouth. May cause nausea, vomiting, and poor appetite.

Dactinomycin (Cosmegen). Given as an injection or through an iv. May cause stomatitis, nausea, vomiting, diarrhea, and poor appetite.

Doxorubicin HCl (Adriamycin). Given as an injection. May cause stomatitis, nausea, vomiting.

Fluorouracil (Fluorouracil). Given through an iv. May cause stomatitis, nausea, vomiting, diarrhea, and poor appetite.

Methotrexate (Methotrexate). Given as an injection, through an iv, or by mouth. May cause stomatitis, nausea, vomiting, abdominal distress, and poor appetite.

Nitrogen Mustard (Mustargen). Given as an injection or through an iv. May cause nausea, vomiting, diarrhea, metallic taste, and poor appetite.

Vinblastine Sulfate (Velban). Given as an injection or through an iv. May cause stomatitis, nausea, vomiting, diarrhea, or constipation, abdominal distress and poor appetite.

Vincristine Sulfate (Oncovin). Given as an injection or through an iv. May cause stomatitis, nausea, vomiting, diarrhea, or constipation, abdominal distress and poor appetite.

Cholesterol Lowering Medication

Cholestyramine (Questran). Diet Recommendations: Do not take with carbonated beverages. May cause taste changes.

Diabetes Medications

Insulin. Follow physician's recommendations for administration. Diet Recommendations: Physician should prescribe a diabetic exchange diet.

Tolbutamide (Orinase). Take at a regular time each day. Diet Recommendations: Avoid alcohol. Physician should prescribe diabetic exchange diet. May cause poor appetite and gastric upset.

Tolazamide (Tolinase). Take at regular time each day as prescribed by physician. Diet Recommendations: Avoid alcohol.

Physician should prescribe diabetic exchange diet. May cause poor appetite and gastric upset.

Diuretics

Furosemide (Lasix). Take with food in the morning. Diet Recommendations: Increase foods high in potassium (oranges, orange juice, bananas, potatoes, tomatoes). Increase foods high in magnesium (milk, yogurt). Consult physician on alcohol. May cause nausea, poor appetite and dizziness. Physician should monitor blood levels of potassium, sodium, magnesium, and calcium.

Hydrochlorothiazide (Hydrodiuril, Oretic). Take with food in the morning. Diet Recommendations: Physician may prescribe a low sodium diet. Increase foods high in potassium (oranges, orange juice, bananas, potatoes, tomatoes). Increase foods high in magnesium (milk, yogurt). Consult physician on alcohol. May cause nausea, poor appetite and dizziness. Physician should monitor blood levels of potassium, sodium, magnesium, and calcium.

Spironlactone (Aldactone). Take with food in the morning. Physician should monitor blood levels of potassium and sodium. May cause drowsiness and confusion.

Heart Medications

Digitalis, Digoxin (Lanoxin). Take with water. Diet Recommendations: Physician may prescribe a low sodium diet. Increase foods high in potassium (oranges, orange juice, bananas, potatoes, tomatoes). May cause poor appetite.

Diltiazem (Cardizem). Take on an empty stomach, one hour before or two to three hours after a meal. Diet Recommendations: Avoid alcohol. May cause nausea and constipation.

Nifedipine (Procardia). Take on an empty stomach, one hour before or two to three hours after a meal. May cause nausea.

Nitroglycerin (Nitrobid, Nitroglyn). Take with water on empty stomach one hour before or two to three hours after a meal. Diet Recommendations: Avoid alcohol. May cause dizziness.

Prazosin HCl (Minipress). Diet Recommendations: Avoid alcohol. May cause constipation and dizziness.

Verapamil HCl (Isoptin). Take on an empty stomach, one hour before or two to three hours after a meal. Diet Recommendations: Avoid alcohol. May cause dizziness and constipation.

Hormones

Estrogen (Premarin). Take with food. Diabetics should be cautious as this medication may elevate blood sugar. May decrease the absorption of the water soluble vitamins. May cause nausea and fluid gain.

Synthroid-Thyroid Preparation (Levothyroxine Sodium). Take on an empty stomach, one hour before or two to three hours after a meal. May cause nausea, gastric upset, and alter appetite.

Laxatives/Stool Softeners

Docusate Calcium (Surfak). Take with water, juice, or milk. Diet Recommendations: Drink plenty of fluids. May cause gas, cramping.

Docusate Sodium (Colace, Doxinate). Do not take at mealtime. Take with water, juice, or milk. Diet Recommendations: Drink plenty of fluids. May cause gas, cramping, and diarrhea.

Phenolphthalein (Ex-Lax, Feen-A-Mint). Do not take at mealtime. Take with water or milk. Diet Recommendations: Drink plenty of fluids. May cause gas and cramping.

Nausea Medication

Bismuth Subsalicylate (Pepto-Bismol). May cause darkening of stool and tongue. Patients on gout, diabetic, or anticoagulant medications, use caution. Contains salicylates. Should not be used by persons known to be allergic to salicylates or aspirin.

Seizure Medications

Phenytoin Sodium (Dilantin). Take with food or milk with gastric upset. Diet Recommendations: Avoid alcohol. May cause taste changes and constipation.

Phenobarbital (Luminal). Take with food or milk with gastric upset. Diet Recommendations: Avoid alcohol.

Medications for Depression

Monoamine Oxidase Inhibitors
Isocarboxazide (Marplan), Phenelzine Sulfate (Nardil), Tranylcypromine Sulfate (Parnate). Take with food. *Important Diet*

Recommendations: Avoid all alcohol. Avoid foods high in pressor amines (i.e., tyramine): sharp and aged cheese (avoid all cheese but cream and cottage cheese), chianti wine particularly red wine, some beers, smoked or pickled fish, salami, pepperoni, summer sausage, chicken or beef livers, Italian broad beans, sour cream, yogurt, soy sauce, bananas, figs, raisins. Avoid an excessive amount of caffeine-containing beverages. May cause headache and severe hypertension if medication is taken with these foods high in pressor amines.

Tricyclic

   Amitriptyline (Elavil), Doxepin HCl (Sinequan, Adapin).   Take with food. Diet Recommendations: Avoid alcohol. May cause an increased appetite for carbohydrate-containing foods. May cause dry mouth.

Pain Relievers

   Acetaminophen (Tylenol, (Datril).   Take on an empty stomach as food delays absorption.
   Acetylsalicylic Acid (Aspirin).   Take with food as medication may cause gastrointestinal upset. Long-term use may cause gastrointestinal bleeding and contribute to iron deficiency anemia. Should not be used by people prone to bleeding or deficient in vitamin K. Diet Recommendations: For long-term use increase food sources of vitamin C (oranges, orange juice, other citrus fruit, green leafy vegetables, cantaloupe, strawberries, broccoli).

Ulcer Medications

   Cimetidine (Tagamet).   Take with food. May cause dizziness, stomach cramps, diarrhea, and confusion.

Diet Management of Symptoms
Caused by Medication

Although many medications have specific symptoms that do accompany the dose, there are steps that can be taken to alleviate these symptoms or make them tolerable. If the symptoms persist after taking these steps, you should contact your physician.

Constipation

1. Increase your fiber intake by consuming raw vegetables and fruits, breads and cereals containing wheat bran.
2. Include at least 8 to 10 glasses of fluid per day.
3. Relax after meals.
4. Use warm or hot liquids to stimulate peristalsis (bowel activity).
5. Exercise to your ability and as allowed by your physician.
6. Avoid the use or overuse of laxatives. If constipation continues to be a problem, consult your physician about a stool softener.

Gas

1. Eat slowly to avoid swallowing air.
2. Avoid gas-producing foods. Some foods that commonly produce gas include: cabbage, cauliflower, dried beans, and peas, and any others that cause you gas.

Diarrhea

1. Avoid the gas-producing vegetables such as cabbage, cauliflower, dried beans, and peas.
2. Use cooked fruits and vegetables rather than raw or fresh.
3. Decrease your intake of the fiber-containing foods such as nuts, seeds, produce with tough skin—apples, pears, grapes, whole-grain bread, and cereals.
4. To replace fluids and potassium losses from diarrhea, use fruit juices and nectars, popsicles, fruit ices, and bananas.

Gastric Upset/Acid Stomach

1. Avoid caffeine-containing beverages. Decaffeinated beverages can be used as tolerated but avoid if increase gastric upset.
2. Avoid alcoholic beverages.
3. Avoid black pepper and chili powder.
4. Avoid highly seasoned, spicy, or fried foods if not tolerated.
5. Small frequent meals may reduce the acidity of the stomach and provide some relief.
6. Avoid any additional foods that increase the acidity of your stomach.

Nausea

1. Eat small frequent meals or snacks.
2. Try dry foods (i.e., toast, crackers).
3. Use cool or warm liquids to get through periods of nausea (i.e., ginger ale, clear soups, gelatin, popsicles, or fruit slushes).
4. Avoid fried or greasy foods while nauseated.
5. Avoid exercising after eating.
6. Change to a clear liquid diet (i.e., ginger ale, clear broths or soups, gelatin, popsicles, or fruit slushes) if nausea persists and report to your physician.

Mouth Irritation

1. If mouth is dry, use mints or lemon drops to stimulate saliva production.
2. Chop, grate or blenderize foods. (Heat foods first then blenderize.)
3. Use foods with cool or warm temperatures rather than extreme temperatures.
4. Avoid acid fruits and fruit juices (such as citrus). Try less acidic fruits and fruit juices such as apple, pear, peach, and banana.
5. Suck on popsicles or frozen juices.
6. Avoid spicy, salty, or coarse foods and alcohol.
7. Soak or marinate foods in liquids for a more tender texture.
8. Eat moist foods, casseroles, macaroni and cheese, yogurt until mouth irritation clears.

Poor Appetite/Weight Loss

1. Eat small meals more frequently to increase your calorie intake. Keep foods available to snack on throughout the day and include a bedtime snack.
2. Eat your favorite foods more often.
3. Add powdered milk to milkshakes, puddings, custards, and casseroles to increase the protein and calorie content of foods.
4. Fortify your milk by adding 1 cup of dry milk to 1 quart of fluid milk. This addition doubles the protein content of the milk.

5. Use sugar, salt, and marinades (if allowed on your diet) to enhance flavors of food.

6. Use additional margarine on foods to add calories.

7. Foods high in carbohydrates are often readily consumed and can add calories to the diet: popsicles, jelly and jam, honey, flavored gelatin, marshmallows, and other candies. (Diabetics consult physician on including simple sugars in diet.)

8. If poor appetite and weight loss continue, consult your physician.

Taste Changes

1. If cooked meat, fish or poultry taste bitter, try these protein-rich alternatives: cheese, tuna or chicken salad, ham or egg salad, luncheon meat, deviled eggs, milkshakes, puddings, custards.

2. If you experience a bitter or metallic taste in your mouth, suck on hard candy, rinse your mouth with mouthwash, or drink fruit juice or ginger ale.

3. To avoid an aftertaste with medication, take with applesauce or crushed pineapple or rinse mouth with mouthwash after taking medication.

If you are on one or more medications that can cause food-drug interactions, you should be evaluated periodically by your physician to determine if your drug therapy *adversely* affects you.

□ *PART III*

Responding to Life Changes

CHAPTER 7

Specific Health Problems

Now that we have reviewed some guidelines for maintaining good health, let's look at some specific health problems. When a specific problem appears many of us are reluctant to call a physician, especially after office hours. Although it is reasonable to wait until usual office hours when possible, you should not hesitate to call when a serious problem occurs or when you aren't sure what to do.

The following suggestions for specific actions when certain common medical problems occur are important to the mature adult. The discussions are not intended to be exhaustive medical consultations, but the Additional Readings on page 307 can supply more detailed discussions of these problems. Remember that each one of us is different, so if you have any questions you should contact your physician.

■ AIDS (ACQUIRED IMMUNODEFICIENCY SYNDROME)

AIDS refers to the disease Acquired Immunodeficiency Syndrome. The first cases were recognized in the United States in 1981. The disease has spread rapidly since then and affects all ages. The death rate when the disease runs its course is 100 percent since there is no known cure. AIDS is spread in several ways, one of which is by sexual contact.

Since 1981, researchers have found that a virus named Human Immunodeficiency Virus (HIV) causes AIDS. There are now an estimated 1 to 2 million persons infected with the virus in the United States. While many people infected with the virus will develop AIDS, some may not. By 1991, it is estimated that over 250,000 persons will have AIDS or will have died from AIDS. The virus attacks the body's cells, especially cells in the blood called T4 Helper cells. These cells are very important in the body's defense against infection and tumors. If the T4 Helper cells are diminished or crippled, the body's ability to defend against infection is lowered. Mild infections, easily handled by normal persons, may cause severe disease. Many of these infections have no available treatment or treatment is not effective because the body's defense is so weakened.

The majority of people who presently have been diagnosed as having AIDS are homosexual or bisexual men. Intravenous drug users, men and women, are the second largest group. The disease is spread by (1) sexual contact (about 80 percent of cases), (2) exposure to infected needles, (3) through contact with AIDS infected blood. For example, the baby of an infected mother may have AIDS. Usual daily contacts have not been shown to cause infection. Even those who live in close contact with AIDS patients do not appear to become infected if there is no sexual contact. Once infected, the disease may develop in several months or not for many years. The actual number of persons who will definitely develop AIDS after infection is not known but has been estimated to be 25 to 50 percent or higher.

The infection may cause no symptoms for many years. The infection may first cause an acute illness with fever, fatigue, headache, and appear as a virus-like illness. Other AIDS victims may after months or years develop fever, weight loss, diarrhea, and swelling of lymph nodes. The most common way in which the actual AIDS illness begins is with pneumonia. It is usually caused by one of the forms of pneumonia which a normal person's body defense would not allow. The victim may first notice diarrhea, abdominal pain, nausea, or vomiting. Some AIDS patients are first affected by severe headache and fever from infection in the brain or spinal canal due to meningitis. Many other problems can happen including the development of malignant tumors. Because there is no cure, these problems gradually worsen until the person dies. Available treatment with drugs is highly experimental and largely ineffective.

Diagnosis depends on detecting problems early, usually in a person who is at higher risk because of sexual habits, exposure to blood transfusions, or infected needles. Blood tests detect evidence of HIV infection, but infection does not mean disease . . . yet. It may take 3 to 6 months for a blood test to become positive. Remember that the tests are not perfect. The only prevention is to avoid putting yourself at high risk.

Treatment depends on the specific problem caused by the infection. Treatment of specific infections is offered when possible and general supportive care is given. Counseling and close observation are needed so that new infections and other medical problems are detected and treated as early as possible.

Prevention involves avoiding those situations that create high risk. The risk in receiving blood products is now improved with newer techniques, but is still present. The entire population should be better informed about safe sex practices. Only through education, beginning with our children and grandchildren, can the spread of this disease be slowed.

ALCOHOL PROBLEMS

Alcoholism is one of the most costly of all problems adults face. Alcohol, like other drugs, can be addictive. The alcohol industry depends on advertising in the media, therefore, television and magazines may portray a biased picture of drinking.

Actually, one third of all Americans don't drink at all. Another third drink only on special occasions. The last third of the population are the alcohol consumers and 10 percent of these are alcoholics.

Alcohol may have devastating effects on the individual and society. Alcohol-related damage costs society almost $100 billion a year and over 100,000 lives. Alcohol is the most frequent cause of preventable birth defects such as mental retardation. America loses almost as many lives each year to alcohol as were lost to battle in all the years of the Vietnam War. Only a small proportion of alcohol-related deaths are from cirrhosis, one of the top 10 causes of death in the country. Accidents, homicides, suicides and medical problems account for tens of thousands of alcohol-related deaths. Since many years of emotional trauma precede the physical consequences, many don't appreciate the extent of the damage. It may be impossible to get an exact estimate of the numbers of deaths that are alcohol related.

Alcohol problems are not purely random occurrences. Genetic factors appear to make a person more likely to develop alcohol problems. Ignored and unchecked, the problem will surely continue to proceed to later generations.

"It will never happen to me," "I don't have a problem," "I'll stop before it gets that bad," or "My drinking doesn't hurt anybody but me" are words often spoken by people who are unable or unwilling to do anything about an alcohol problem that already exists. The self-deception commonly known as "denial" presents the major obstacle to recovery. The truth is that anyone can get into trouble with alcohol. Some people are more at risk than others. The drinker is no more able to avoid an alcohol problem than one could avoid a heart attack, diabetes, or cancer. Like those diseases, however, prevention can minimize the risk of future problems. Family members also experience denial. By "enabling" the person with the problem, the family protects the person they love from the consequences of his or her behavior and destroys any realistic opportunity for constructive intervention which leads to help.

The road toward dependence implies that to become a problem, alcohol needs to first become important in the life of its victim. In spite of its devastating consequences alcohol becomes too important for the problem drinker to give up. Since alcohol seems to alleviate some problems the family may not understand its important causative role. The self-destructive spiral of late stage alcoholism becomes evident as alcohol is consumed in an attempt to cushion the pain of previous drinking.

The best way to get help is to avoid problems in the first place. For a person who has a family background of alcohol problems adoption of an abstinent lifestyle represents the safest choice.

Help is available universally in some form. Alcoholics Anonymous (A.A.) provides the most effective and inexpensive therapy, but sometimes physical addiction and medical complications require medical help from a physician or hospital specializing in addiction. The book *Alcoholics Anonymous* can be purchased at any A.A. group and should be required reading for one who worries about his own or someone else's drinking.

■ ALZHEIMER'S DISEASE, MEMORY LOSS, AND DEMENTIA

Memory allows us to retain information about past events; memory is important for our daily activities and interactions with other persons. Many of us think of memory loss as a part of old age and loss of mental function. Many persons have great concerns that any memory failures may mean the early onset of Alzheimer's disease. When should we become concerned about our memory failures? How do we tell the difference between everyday forgetfulness and serious memory failure? There is no definite answer but researchers do have some suggestions.

If you are otherwise healthy, occasional forgetfulness or failure of memory should not be of severe concern. Young adults probably have occasional memory failures but are less concerned that this represents serious memory loss. There is evidence that most mature adults do have some changes in memory with at least occasional memory failure, especially after the middle years. This alone is not considered abnormal and it does not interfere with activities in our daily lives.

Memory failures that are frequent or interfere with daily activity are more cause for concern. Frequent forgetting of appointments, names, places, or recent events can interfere with daily function. If these memory failures happen suddenly or become frequent then further medical evaluation is needed. Loss of memory may be one of the first signs of overall decrease in mental activity and mental function of the brain. If this process continues the medical term is *dementia*. Dementia refers to an overall decrease in mental activity and mental function. There is a decrease in the higher intellectual functions of the brain. This affects areas such as judgment, memory, language, behavior, and physical activities.

The most common cause of dementia is Alzheimer's disease, which has no known specific cause or cure. But there are some other medical problems which can cause dementia or make dementia worse. Some of them are treatable if detected early. If you notice memory failure which begins to interfere with daily activity in yourself or a family member, you should discuss the problem with your physician.

Alzheimer's disease may begin after age 40 but usually is diagnosed after age 65. There is no definite evidence that having a family member with Alzheimer's disease greatly increases the risk that other family members will be affected.

Memory failure is usually the first sign. This is one reason for the anxiety many persons feel when they notice minor memory failures. Memory failures may not be noticed over months or even years. Over this period of time, there may be gradual changes and deterioration in behavior. For example, previous thoughtfulness, warmth, and emotions may lessen. Reasoning power, judgment, and language may gradually deteriorate. Decisions in business or personal life may become more difficult and may not be made as wisely. Daily activities eventually become more difficult, such as driving a car. Later on basic activities such as dressing and eating become more difficult. Loss of control of bowels or bladder may occur. The person may become severely limited and bedridden.

At first, the changes may be very subtle and difficult to identify. At this point, decisions may be made by a person which are not in their own best interest. At this time these actions may bring anger from family and friends because the true problem is not yet evident. Eventually the problems dealing with daily activity become so great that the problem of dementia is apparent to others.

At some point other responsible persons such as a spouse or family may need to assume more responsibility in advice and decision making. This can be a difficult time. As the disease progresses, it eventually becomes easier for others to make decisions. Until this time comes, there is no easy answer for family and friends. Much care and support is needed.

Tests include a computed tomographic (CT) scan of the head, blood tests, and other studies. There is no easily available, specific test that can absolutely diagnose Alzheimer's disease. There are some tests that detect early changes in mental activity and function which may be useful.

Other medical problems, emotional stress, and psychological problems can greatly aggravate many of the problems of Alzheimer's disease. An illness may make all of the symptoms and signs of dementia and Alzheimer's disease suddenly worsen. Treatment of any underlying illness may help a return to the previous level. If there is a sudden change or worsening in a person who has dementia then it is worthwhile to look for *another* medical problem that might be treatable. For example, an infection can make a person with dementia seem to become much worse. Treatment of the infection may result in improvement in dementia. Talk with your physician.

Possible treatments: Once other medical problems have been evaluated and treated, there is no other specific treatment for Alzheimer's disease. The course may be rapid over months but more commonly slowly worsens over years. There may be a gradual deterioration in the ability of the person to handle self-care. There may be periods of slight improvement which last months or years. In many cases, it becomes impossible for the person to continue to live at home alone or with a spouse or family. When this happens, it may be necessary to receive care in a nursing home or similar facility. Such a facility may be better able to care for all of the needs of the person. This is undoubtedly a difficult decision for a spouse or family.

It is important to provide an environment that prevents problems which might aggravate the loss of mental ability. Prevention and control of other medical problems, good nutrition and cleanliness, exercise when possible, and reasonable emotional support are the goals of treatment at this point.

■ ANEMIA

Anemia refers to a lower than normal level of hemoglobin measured in the blood. Although it is common to feel fatigue and tiredness, a blood test is needed to discover anemia. Guidelines to suggest anemia include a blood test which shows a hemoglobin of less than 12 grams/dl in a female or less than 14 grams/dl in a male. However, each person is different and other medical problems may greatly affect how the level of hemoglobin is interpreted. For example, some forms of arthritis and some forms of kidney disease commonly cause a lower hemoglobin than normal as part of the problem.

Discussion, examination, and testing will be planned to be sure that there is no abnormal loss of blood which might create anemia. Tests will be planned to be sure that the body is making blood properly. Your physician can guide you so that the proper diagnosis and treatment can be given with the least number of tests required.

■ ANXIETY

A troubled, worried feeling or fear of what may happen in the future is common in normal persons. These are normal reactions to events and stress in our everyday life. Usually these feelings are temporary and do not interfere with our daily lives on a regular basis.

If these feelings of uneasiness, worry, and fear of what may happen become severe or constant or when they interfere with daily activity, further evaluation is useful. The feelings may come on suddenly and produce severe anxiety with palpitations, dizziness, shortness of breath, and sweating. Anxiety over a specific event or activity may be severe or limiting. Some persons develop severe anxiety after injuries in an accident or catastrophe.

If the anxiety becomes limiting or interferes with daily activity then it is best to have further evaluation. Talk with your physician. After discussion and examination other medical problems can be eliminated. Then plans can be made to control the anxiety so that it is no longer limiting. This often includes evaluation by a psychiatrist or clinical psychologist as well as medication to control the symptoms.

■ ARTHRITIS

One of the most common causes of pain around joints and muscles is arthritis—inflammation in and around the joints. Over 100 kinds of arthritis affect 30 million Americans. About half of those over age 65 have significant arthritis problems, but arthritis is not at all limited to older persons. Some of the most limiting kinds of arthritis are most common in women and men just when they are most productive in work and family. Arthritis *can* be controlled in the majority of persons. Early diagnosis and proper treatment can change a severely limiting situation into one that is manageable.

Arthritis can develop gradually or suddenly. There is usually pain and stiffness in the joints, and there may be swelling. At times the joints may be warm or red. When the hands are affected, there may be difficulty with daily activities such as buttons, washing dishes, using tools, and even eating. When the knees are involved, there may be difficulty in standing and walking. Arthritis in the shoulders may make it difficult to dress, especially in the mornings when stiffness may be prominent.

In some kinds of arthritis such as osteoarthritis, the problems are limited to pain in the joints. In rheumatoid arthritis there may be deformities of the joints, fever, weight loss, and severe fatigue. There may also be inflammation around the heart, lungs, and eyes in rheumatoid arthritis. Some forms of arthritis may be life-threatening.

If pain or swelling in the joints has no apparent reason or lasts longer than a few days, it would be worthwhile to ask your physician for advice. Pain or stiffness that results from excessive use such as in yardwork, sports activities, or other "weekend" activity usually goes away after a few days or more. Pain or swelling that is persistent or recurrent should be evaluated.

Treatment depends on the kind of arthritis. Usually moist heat (or at times ice!) is applied to the joints for 20 to 30 minutes, twice daily, along with an exercise program. Exercises keep the joints flexible and limber and strengthen the muscles. Stronger muscles are important to give the joints more support but arthritis commonly makes muscles weaker. Exercises are among the most important parts of the treatment for arthritis.

Medications may also be helpful in many kinds of arthritis. The most commonly used are a group of medications called anti-inflammatory drugs. Cortisone-like medications are the strongest anti-inflammatory drugs. These medications can dramatically improve joint pain and swelling. In fact, when they were discovered it was hoped that a cure had been found for arthritis. But it was found that they also had side effects which may be serious. As a result, other drugs were used which may decrease inflammation but do not have as many side effects as the cortisone-like drugs. These are called the noncortisone or nonsteroid anti-inflammatory drugs. They are not as potent as the cortisone derivatives. Many are available including aspirin and ibuprofen. Over the years, many other newer drugs have been developed to try to improve control of the inflammation of arthritis with as few side effects as possible. It is not possible to predict in an individual which medication will be the most effective or have the fewest side effects. A trial of a number of different medications in this group may be necessary to find the most effective one. Your physician can help you find the drug that is best for you.

The potential side effects of most nonsteroid anti-inflammatory drugs are similar. Even though most patients have no side effects, it is important to always be on the lookout for any unwanted effects; then the medication can usually be stopped and side effects minimized. The most common side effects are nausea, indigestion, heartburn, and upset stomach. Ulcers in the stomach and intestine, intestinal bleeding and abnormalities of the liver and kidney may occur. There are many other potential side effects, some of which can be treated by stopping the medication or other simple measures.

In arthritis treatment as well as in other problems, the benefits of treatment should outweigh the risks. The chances for improvement should be greater than the risks of side effects from the medications. Most effective treatments in arthritis have potential side effects. If you have pain, swelling, and stiffness in the joints from arthritis then your physician can guide you to the treatments that offer the most benefit with the least potential for side effects.

In some kinds of more severe arthritis such as rheumatoid arthritis, there is another group of medications which may be used. These medications are intended to suppress the arthritis at a more basic level. They take longer to work and have potential side effects but often give excellent relief. The potential side effects can usually be controlled by careful observation on the part of patient and physician.

Most kinds of arthritis can be controlled. A reasonable goal is to expect to be able to be comfortable and to do most daily activities in reasonable comfort. In some cases, your physician may ask that you be seen by an arthritis specialist, a rheumatologist.

(See also *osteoarthritis, rheumatoid arthritis.*)

■ ASTHMA

Asthma refers to spells of wheezing, tightness in the chest, shortness of breath, or cough. The feelings usually occur intermittently and can result in a severe illness. The spells can follow an infection, occur with allergies or after exercise. The episodes may also happen in persons who already have other lung diseases. Exposure to chemicals, gases, and dusts may bring on an episode.

During the episode, there may be severe shortness of breath, wheezing, gasping for air, and coughing, or the episode may be milder with only coughing. Medical evaluation is needed. Your physician will look for underlying causes of the asthma and remove any possible specific factors possible. Medications are available that control the acute attacks and may help prevent or control future attacks. In some cases, your physician may ask that you be seen by a specialist such as a pulmonary (lung) specialist or an allergist.

■ BACK PAIN

Almost everyone will suffer from back pain sometime. Lower back pain is one of the major causes of missed work days in this country. Most back pain is limited in duration and usually is caused by an injury such as an automobile accident, a fall, or heavy lifting. However, some individuals develop severe back pain which may become constant and severely limiting.

The spine is a complex structure made up of vertebral bones separated from each other by discs which allow motion. Strong, thick ligaments and muscles keep the discs and vertebrae aligned and prevent the spinal cord from injury. Also, nerve fibers are present leaving the spinal cord and traveling to supply the body. Small joints are present and allow the bony vertebrae to move as a unit.

Most back pain is due to *strain*, especially in the lower (lumbar) spine. This lumbar strain is usually limited in duration and is often found to be caused by an injury such as an automobile accident, a fall, or improper or heavy lifting. The severe pain usually goes away after 7 to 10 days and is helped by rest, application of moist heat, and at times medications for pain. After the pain goes away, a regular exercise program may help to prevent or decrease future attacks of pain.

In some persons, these episodes of pain become more frequent and pain may become constant and severely limiting. This can be a difficult problem to control. Tests are usually done to be sure no other problem is present which might be treated in other ways. A program of moist heat, exercises, and medications often gives improvement even if there is not complete relief of pain. Medications used include anti-inflammatory drugs, muscle relaxants, and occasional pain medication. Physical therapy can help with a regular program of heat and exercises. Persons who are able to maintain a regular exercise program often find more improvement than those who for various reasons cannot do exercises for the back regularly.

Lumbar Disc Disease is a common cause of lower back pain. The discs most commonly affected are those at the lower part of the lumbar spine. Injury is the most common precipitating cause. At times, there may be no important injury. Some persons have had earlier injuries leading up to the final disc rupture or may have a weakness in their supporting ligaments. Back pain due to disc rupture or herniation is often severe and may be worsened by coughing, sneezing, or bending. If a nerve root is under pressure, the person will feel pain down the leg and often into the foot. Numbness and burning in the same area of the leg is common. It is as if "hot water was poured down the leg."

On examination, the physician may find muscle spasm, difficulty with walking, and pain in the back when the straightened leg is raised. X-rays of the lower spine are often not very helpful. A computed tomographic (CT) scan of the lumbar spine or a magnetic resonance imaging (MRI) study may help make a diagnosis. At times, a myelogram in which dye is injected into the spinal canal is needed to make the proper diagnosis. Other tests are available that can detect abnormalities of the nerve supply and conduction of the nerves from the spine into the legs.

Treatment includes rest, usually in bed, and medications to control the pain and muscle spasm. Traction may help at times. Some persons improve with these measures alone. If there is no improvement or there are frequent recurrences, surgery may offer relief.

Arthritis is another common cause of back pain. Osteoarthritis is the most common type of arthritis and a frequent cause of back pain. This is especially common in older people. Spurs may form near the spine as a result of osteoarthritis. A nerve may be "pinched" if one of these spurs is in a strategic position. X-rays of the spine will usually show the changes of osteoarthritis, but the amount of arthritis present on x-ray may be more or less severe than the pain seems to be.

Treatment for this cause of back pain includes moist heat, proper rest, exercises, and anti-inflammatory medications. Muscle relaxants and pain medications may be needed. It is good to try to keep the use of strong pain medications such as narcotics to a minimum. Physical therapy in a regular program of heat and exercises is helpful.

Osteoporosis (thinning of the bones) may cause severe back pain. If the bones become weak enough, minor strain or injury may result in a compression fracture in a vertebral bone. (See Figure 6 on page 55) This is most common in the lower (lumbar) part of the spine. The pain may be severe and usually slowly improves over 3 to

6 weeks. Osteoporosis is most common in women after menopause. The diagnosis of compression fracture is made on x-ray. Other tests can diagnose osteoporosis. Treatment of the osteoporosis is used to try to prevent future fractures. Treatment of the compression fracture usually consists of rest, pain medications, and a gradual increase in activity. (See page 55.)

A form of arthritis found most commonly in men is *ankylosing spondylitis*. The back pain is usually gradual in onset over years with stiffness in the morning on arising. It may result in limited spine movement. The diagnosis is made after discussion, examination, x-ray of the back, and blood tests. A high risk for this disease appears to be genetic. Ninety percent of persons with ankylosing spondylitis have a blood test positive for HLA-B27 antigen.

Scoliosis (curvature of the spine) is common in our population and may be a cause of back pain. Inflammation in the muscles and soft tissues of the back may cause pain when *fibrositis* is present (see the discussion of *Fibrositis* on page 186). *Cancer or infection* in or near the spine may cause back pain. Specific tests will be ordered when these problems are suspected.

Pain may be felt in the back even though the cause of the pain may be elsewhere. This is an example of *referred pain*. For instance, pain may be felt in the back from an ulcer in the stomach. Many other internal organ problems may cause back pain. Your physician can guide your own situation. Because of the many possible causes of back pain a thorough examination is required of the back, extremities, abdomen, pelvis, and blood vessels. This might be followed by blood tests, x-rays, CT scan, MRI, myelogram, and other studies.

■ BELL'S PALSY

Bell's palsy results from weakness or paralysis of the facial nerve which is responsible for facial motion. This is almost always on one side rather than both sides of the face. The cause is viral invasion of the nerve. There is usually pain in the area of the ear but, on occasion, no pain is present. There may be increased tearing and change in taste as well. Treatment is usually with medication but on occasion an operation is required. Special electrical diagnostic tests, and sometimes special x-rays, are done which point to the location of the block and help predict the future course. In the majority of cases, the nerve regains most of its function in 6 to 10 weeks.

■ BRONCHITIS (ACUTE)

Acute bronchitis usually starts as a cough with production of sputum which may be thick and yellow. Fever and fatigue may be present. Wheezing and shortness of breath may be present, especially in those who smoke cigarettes or have chronic bronchitis.

Tests which might be ordered include a chest x-ray to be sure there is no pneumonia present and blood tests to measure oxygen levels in the blood called arterial blood gases.

Possible treatments include antibiotics. Cigarette smoking should be stopped. Medications called bronchodilators may be used if wheezing is prominent. The purpose of these medications is to decrease the narrowing of the bronchial tubes and allow easier breathing. At times, especially when other lung disease is present, oxygen may be prescribed.

■ BRONCHITIS (CHRONIC)

In chronic bronchitis, there is a cough with sputum (phlegm) for an extended period without another cause. The cough is usually worse in the morning after arising. As the chronic bronchitis worsens, the cough lasts longer into the day and night. Wheezing and shortness of breath may be present as the disease worsens.

More rapid or difficult breathing, especially with activity, becomes worse as the disease progresses. The amount of sputum may increase. Later, usually after years, there may be bluish discoloration of the fingernails because of changes in the oxygen in the blood. Colds or other respiratory infections often result in more severe illnesses such as acute bronchitis or pneumonia. The periods of severe cough and shortness of breath gradually get closer together so that eventually these problems may be continuous.

Tests which may be ordered include chest x-ray, blood tests including oxygen and carbon dioxide levels, lung function tests, and other tests. The tests are to exclude other causes of the problem and to help decide the severity of the chronic bronchitis.

Possible treatments include quitting smoking and medications such as bronchodilators in the oral form or aerosol sprays. Antibiotics may be used for acute infections. Oxygen therapy may be required. Admission to a hospital for more intensive treatment may be needed at times.

■ BURSITIS

Bursitis is one cause of pain around a joint which can be very severe and limiting. A bursa lies outside of a joint and is a specially lubricated area through which tendons and muscles move more smoothly. When bursitis is present, there is pain on any movement of the muscles or tendons. The first sensation of bursitis may be pain near a joint that worsens when the joint is moved or with pressure on the joint. The pain may be mild or severe and may last from a few days to months or even years. The areas most commonly affected are the shoulders and hips. At times, certain activities such as repetitive movements of an arm in one direction or in one activity (such as hammering) may seem to trigger the attack of bursitis.

There is pain with pressure in the area, and swelling and warmth may be present as well. The pain is often most severe with pressure on the front or side of the shoulder or at the side of the hip. Other areas which may be affected are the front of the knees (housemaid's knees), the buttocks (weaver's bottom), and around the elbows.

If the pain is severe, you should see your physician. Other more serious conditions must be eliminated. X-rays and blood tests may be taken to help guide the treatment.

Treatment usually includes heat application such as a heating pad or warm shower. Massage of the area may be helpful. The involved joint should have gradual increase in exercise and activity as pain allows. Your physician may suggest an anti-inflammatory medication to help decrease the pain and allow more movement. If the pain is severe or persistent, an injection into the bursa with a cortisone derivative may be given. This injection often gives quick and effective relief. It is important to remember that bursitis usually improves and is not usually a serious condition over a long period.

■ CANCER

Breast Cancer. The incidence of breast cancer appears to be steadily increasing. It is estimated that by the year 2000, one of 10 American women will develop breast cancer sometime during their lifetime. Despite the rising incidence of breast cancer, the mortality rate has risen much more slowly. This suggests that the likelihood of surviving breast cancer is better than in the past. It would appear that this improvement in survival is secondary to screening, early detection, and better initial treatment.

Breast cancer can occur in women of all ages, although the risk steadily increases with age, peaking between ages 50 and 60. Breast cancer in a sister or mother, especially prior to menopause, increases the risk of developing breast cancer by three to four times. Benign breast disease, estrogen treatment for postmenopausal symptoms, obesity, breast feeding, number of pregnancies, and diet have not been proven to significantly increase the incidence of breast cancer. Early pregnancy (before the age of 18) may have some protective effect. However, most of the readers will find it too late for themselves and unacceptable for their daughters.

Breast cancer usually is first detected as a painless lump in the breast. This lump tends to be firm and may or may not be moveable. Advanced disease may be associated with pain, thickening or redness of the overlying skin, or lumps in the underarm area (axilla). If a breast lump is discovered, this should be immediately evaluated by a physician. If the lump feels suspicious, the physician will order a mammogram to document malignancy and rule out other malignancy that cannot be felt. Unfortunately, the mammogram may miss 10 to 20 percent of all malignancies. Therefore, any lump that feels suspicious or has an abnormal mammogram, should have a biopsy (surgical removal for pathologic examination).

Breast cancer treatment continues to improve. In the last 15 years, we have seen significant changes in management of localized breast cancer. Acceptable treatment requires removal of the tumor and the immediately surrounding breast tissue and a sampling of the lymph nodes in the underarm (axilla). This is usually achieved by a modified radical mastectomy or a wide excision of the cancer with axillary lymph node sampling and radiation therapy. A modified radical mastectomy is the surgical removal of the entire breast and axillary lymph nodes. A wide excision (lumpectomy, tilectomy, quadrantectomy) removes the breast tissue near the cancer. At the time of wide excision, several of the axillary lymph nodes are removed for pathologic examination. The remainder of the involved breast and usually the axilla will require radiation therapy. Not all breast cancers are acceptable candidates for wide excision with radiation therapy. Each person is different and each case must be treated as unique.

Evaluation of the primary breast tumor and axillary lymph nodes helps determine the probability of recurrence of the breast cancer. Researchers have shown that involvement of the axillary lymph nodes increases the risk of recurrence almost twofold. More recently, determination of DNA content in tumor cells has been proven helpful to predict risk of recurrence. It is recommended that all premenopausal women with axillary lymph nodes involved receive six months of adjuvant chemotherapy. This has been shown to improve their survival. In the postmenopausal woman, this is not quite as clear. Those postmenopausal women who have cancers that may respond to hormonal treatment are usually given the anti-estrogen Tamoxifen (Nolvadex). Other postmenopausal women with cancers are placed on six months of chemotherapy on an individual basis.

Women with breast cancer and without spread to axillary lymph nodes have not been treated with adjuvant chemotherapy in the past. Recently several clinical trials have shown a survival benefit for those women receiving short courses of chemotherapy following surgery. This is controversial with no definite resolution. Adjuvant chemotherapy in women with negative axillary nodes should be determined on an individual basis. Size of the tumor and other factors such as DNA content will probably be important in making these decisions.

Those women with breast cancer that has spread beyond the confines of surgery or local radiation may eventually die from their malignancy. However, breast cancer is considered a disease responsive to chemotherapy, hormonal manipulation, or radiation therapy. It is possible to improve the quality and many times the quantity of life with these treatments. We have all seen the occasional patient with disseminated breast cancer who has enjoyed many years of complete remission with treatment as simple as hormones.

Cancer of the Colon.   Cancer of the colon and rectum can occur in any age group, although it is much more common after age 55. Colorectal cancer is the second most common cancer in the United States. It is estimated that about 151,000 new cases occurred in 1989 with about 61,300 deaths due to colorectal cancer. The frequency of this cancer varies throughout the world. For example, it tends to occur more often in industrialized countries such as the United States with diets low in fiber and high in fat content.

There are several acquired and inherited conditions which increase the risk of colorectal cancer. The most common situation is in those persons with colorectal polyps. These are benign (noncancer) tumors arising from the inside lining of the colon and rectum. Polyps which are larger than 2 centimeters in size have a higher potential for malignant change in the future. Having a colon polyp once makes that person at higher risk for future polyps.

Ulcerative colitis is an inflammatory disease of the colon and rectum which occurs in young adulthood. Severe cases lasting more than 10 years have a higher chance of developing colorectal cancer.

Most cases of colorectal cancer are not inherited, but there are some conditions which run in families that result in a much higher risk of colorectal cancer.

There may be few early symptoms or feelings in colorectal cancer. This means that the cancer may be quite advanced before the development of symptoms. Pain is not very common unless the cancer causes obstruction of the intestine or spreads to surrounding tissues. Before the development of pain, it is more common to notice change in bowel habits or blood in the stool. The changes in bowel habits most commonly noticed are increasing constipation, narrowed size of the stool, or pain with bowel movements. Cancers of the colon may also at times cause mild diarrhea.

The most common sign in colorectal cancer is blood in the stool. Bleeding from other causes such as hemorrhoids, benign polyps, and other problems are much more common than colorectal cancer. However, rectal bleeding must always be assumed to be colorectal carcinoma until proven otherwise. Many persons with far advanced colorectal carcinoma report having noticed rectal bleeding over a long period of time which had been thought to be due only to hemorrhoids.

Unexplained abdominal discomfort, bleeding from the rectum or in the stool, or a change in bowel habits should be reported to your physician. These changes suggest the need for a colon examination. This can be done by barium enema (x-ray of the large intestine) or colonoscopy in which a fiberoptic flexible tube is used to directly examine the entire colon. Colonoscopy has the advantage of being able to biopsy suspicious lesions and remove benign polyps at the time of the examination. If a barium enema is used, then the lower portion of the colon is usually examined by sigmoidoscopy which uses a fiberoptic tube to directly examine this area.

Surgery is the most effective treatment for colorectal cancer. Of patients found to have colorectal cancer, 75 percent will be able to be operated for cure; 50 percent or more may be cured of the cancer at the time of surgery.

A common fear in colorectal cancer is that all patients who have surgery must have a colostomy. In fact, only cancers occurring very close to the anus will require a permanent colostomy. This probably accounts for less than 10 percent of cases of colorectal cancer. Most surgery requires removal of the cancer and a portion of the surrounding intestine and supporting structures.

Despite excellent surgical techniques, not all colorectal cancer can be cured by surgery. Examination of the cancer by the pathologist after surgery helps to identify those persons who are at higher risk of developing recurrence. Research has attempted to show whether the addition of radiation treatment or chemotherapy will improve the cure rate. In some patients with rectal cancers, there has been a small survival benefit by the addition of radiation and chemotherapy.

Twenty to 25 percent of colorectal cancers will be found to have spread into other organs when first diagnosed or at surgery. Unless the life expectancy is very short, surgery is often performed to prevent obstruction of the intestine. Many patients with what is thought to be "incurable colorectal cancer" will have a slow course which will allow survival for a few years or longer if obstruction is prevented.

Chemotherapy has been of limited benefit in treating those colorectal cancers which have spread to other organs. Response rates have been quite low. Newer combinations of treatment may increase the response rate in the future.

Cancer of the Kidney and Bladder. The most common cancer of the urinary tract is cancer of the prostate which is discussed on page 213. Renal (kidney) and bladder cancers are the next most common in men and women.

There may be no unusual feelings or signs of these cancers. The diagnosis may be made after a routine test of urine in which blood is discovered. (See page 230 for discussion of blood in urine.) There are no specific symptoms which suggest cancer of the kidney or bladder. To detect these problems early, it is important that any sign or change in the urinary tract be noticed. This includes frequency of urination, burning or pain on urination, or a feeling of urgency to urinate. Blood noticed in the urine or a change in the pattern of urination (such as a sudden increase in nighttime urination) may all be important signs. As in other problems, the sooner the diagnosis is made, the more effective treatment will be.

After discussion and examination, tests will be planned for more specific diagnosis. These tests include IVP (intravenous pyelogram), computed tomographic (CT) scan, and magnetic resonance imaging (MRI). Other blood and urine tests will be planned. Biopsy is often used to confirm the diagnosis. Once a specific diagnosis is made, proper treatment can be planned.

A 75-year-old man was recently seen after a routine examination found blood in the urine. Direct examination of the bladder in the office with cystoscopy found a bladder cancer. Surgery performed through the penis allowed complete removal of the cancer. The patient is now seen at 4- to 6-month intervals to be sure the cancer does not return.

Cancer of the Lung. Lung cancer is the most common cancer in the United States. In 1989, there will be about 155,000 new cases of lung cancer and about 142,000 deaths related to lung cancer. Cigarette smoking is directly related to the rise in lung cancer. Despite the high incidence of lung cancer and known risk factors, screening for this disease has not been shown to be very effective. We need to emphasize prevention by eliminating cigarette smoking.

A cough is the most common symptom in patients with lung cancer. The cough is persistent and may or may not be productive of sputum. A cough that produces blood always requires immediate evaluation. Any persistent cough or change in chronic cough should be further evaluated by your physician.

Shortness of breath occurs frequently with lung cancer. This can be caused by blockage of the bronchial tubes when wheezing may be present. It can also be caused by the accumulation of fluid in the chest cavity as a result of the cancer.

Pain may occur in the chest area. This pain is usually an aching sensation which may be made worse by deep breathing, coughing, or sneezing. Other symptoms may include hoarseness, difficulty swallowing, loss of weight, or signs caused by spread of the cancer to other areas of the body.

Lung cancer is usually detected on chest x-ray. Once detected, attempts are made to make a specific diagnosis and to determine if the cancer has spread. A computed tomography (CT) scan of the chest may confirm the presence of the cancer and look for evidence or spread of the cancer in the chest. Depending on the location of the tumor, bronchoscopy or needle biopsy may be planned. In bronchoscopy, a small flexible fiberoptic tube is passed through the nose into the bronchial tubes. This may show the cancer and allow a biopsy. In some cases, a very thin needle may be passed through the chest wall directly into the tumor guided by x-ray to allow a biopsy. It should be noted that if these biopsies are negative, it does not eliminate the presence of cancer.

If a diagnosis has not been made by bronchoscopy or needle biopsy, then an open biopsy may be planned. Usually the middle of the chest (mediastinum) is evaluated first and if no diagnosis is made, the surgery may be extended to open the chest (thoracotomy) and remove the tumor.

Treatment for lung cancer depends on the cell type (histologic type) found on biopsy and the stage or spread of the cancer. There are several common cell types of lung cancer. Small cell carcinoma is usually found when already in a late stage. It usually has already spread beyond the confines of surgical treatment. Use of chemotherapy has been accepted for over 15 years in small cell carcinoma. The response rates are good with an improvement in the duration of survival which formerly had often been only 6 to 18 weeks after the diagnosis. Survival for two years in up to 35 percent of cases has been noted with some treatments which may include radiation therapy and chemotherapy.

Cancer of the Pancreas. The pancreas is an organ located in the back portion of the upper abdomen. It produces digestive juices which are excreted into the small intestine. The pancreas also produces hormones including insulin. When cancer develops in the pancreas the 5-year survival rate is less than 5 percent. This poor outlook is due to the late detection of the malignancy. At this time, there is no practical and effective way to screen to detect early cancer of the pancreas.

Weight loss is the most common symptom of patients with pancreatic cancer. Abdominal pain is usually the reason that persons seek medical attention. The pain is often described as "gnawing" in the upper abdomen and may radiate into the back. Although the pain occurs in the area in which one might feel pain from a peptic ulcer or from gallbladder disease, the pain is usually not affected by eating food. Blockage of the bile flow by the cancer may cause jaundice. This can also cause lighter, clay-colored stools, dark urine, and itching. Less frequent symptoms of pancreatic cancer may include change in bowel habits, fever, nausea, and vomiting.

Computed tomographic (CT) scan of the abdomen is often best to detect an abnormal mass in the pancreas. This method may also be used to guide a needle biopsy of the mass to confirm the diagnosis. Sonogram is another examination which is painless and may help detect abnormal masses in the pancreas.

Only a small portion of patients are diagnosed early enough to be cured by surgery. The vast majority will die from this cancer. Quality of life should be the most important factor in planning treatment. Radiation to the pancreas may help relieve pain, jaundice, and other symptoms. Nerve blocks or other procedures are occasionally required for pain relief. Chemotherapy has had limited value in this malignancy.

Cancer of the Uterus. Cancer of the endometrium (inner lining of the uterus) is more common after age 35. There may be no feelings or signs. There may be changes in the menstrual period or irregular vaginal bleeding. Pap smears may occasionally assist in the detection of endometrial cancer. Usually a sample of the lining of the uterus is needed for diagnosis. This can be done by several tests including endometrial biopsy, dilation and curettage, or other methods.

Treatment is effective if there is early diagnosis. This requires care to report any changes in vaginal bleeding. Don't wait for other signs to appear. Maintain your regular schedule of examinations as discussed in Chapter 2. Then you can have peace of mind that you are taking reasonable actions to control this cause of cancer.

Cancer of the Cervix. (See *pap smear*, page 191.)

Cancer of the Vagina. Cancer of the vagina is becoming less common. There is no early discomfort. There may be spotting or vaginal bleeding, especially after intercourse. Routine pelvic examination and pap smear are important for early detection of this cancer. This is often an aggressive cancer and requires immediate evaluation and proper treatment.

■ CARPAL TUNNEL SYNDROME

Carpal tunnel syndrome is a common cause of pain, numbness and tingling in the thumb, index, and middle fingers. The pain and numbness may extend to the forearm or the entire hand. Often the discomfort is worse at night, while driving a car, or with certain positions of the wrists. The feeling is sometimes described as if the hand "went to sleep." The pain or numbness is often improved after movement of the wrist.

The carpal tunnel syndrome is caused by pressure on the median nerve as it passes through the wrist's carpal tunnel. Any process that causes swelling in this small area will create pressure on the nerve. Arthritis, injury, diabetes mellitus, pregnancy, underactive thyroid gland, and other medical problems may cause carpal tunnel syndrome.

The diagnosis is made after discussion and examination. Tests of the nerve as it passes through the wrist may show the cause of the problem. It is important that any underlying cause is found if possible.

Treatment of the underlying problem and a simple splint to be used at night is often effective. Occasionally a local injection to the area gives relief. If there is not improvement or if wasting of the muscles of the hand happens then surgery may be needed.

■ CATARACTS

A cataract is a clouding of the lens inside the eye. Just like a smudge on the lens of the camera will cause a blurred image on the film, so will a cataract cause blurred vision in the eye. Most people will develop cataracts as they age. The age at which a cataract develops in a given individual usually cannot be predicted, but the tendency to develop cataracts runs in families or may occur after an injury to the eye. If the cataract causes difficulty reading, driving a car, or interferes with a person's lifestyle, removal of the cloudy lens should be considered.

A cataract must be removed surgically. The surgery is done as an outpatient and, in most cases, under local anesthesia. Your ophthalmologist can provide further information regarding cataract surgery.

■ CHEST PAIN OR CHEST DISCOMFORT

It is a good thing that so many of us are now aware that discomfort, indigestion or pain that is felt in the chest, neck, jaw, or arm may be caused by a heart attack. This knowledge has alerted many persons to seek proper medical care in time to prevent further serious illness and death from heart attack.

It turns out that there are many other causes of discomfort in the chest which are very common and *not* caused by heart disease. One of the most important decisions in the case of many hospital patients is whether their chest discomfort is caused by heart disease, especially coronary heart disease. For if the cause is in fact coronary heart disease, it is a serious illness and requires treatment to prevent further disease and death. On the other hand, there are some causes of chest pain which are not serious at all and can be ignored!

The problem is how to tell the difference. Many times even after many discussions and routine tests it is difficult for specialists to tell if chest discomfort is caused by coronary heart disease. But now tests are available to tell in almost every situation whether the main cause of the chest discomfort is from coronary heart disease. If coronary heart disease and a few other serious causes of chest discomfort can be ruled out, then it may be possible to be reassured that the chest discomfort will not cause further serious problems.

It is extremely important to tell whether chest discomfort is from coronary heart disease as well as some other less common but serious causes of chest discomfort. The best advice is don't try to guess the cause of your own chest discomfort. It is sometimes difficult for expert cardiologists to tell the cause!

■ CORONARY HEART DISEASE

Coronary heart disease may be felt as discomfort in the chest—feeling pressure, tightness, dull pain, squeezing, heaviness, aching, indigestion, burning or other similar sensations especially when you walk, exert yourself, have a large meal or have strong emotion. The discomfort may seem to move (radiate) toward the neck, jaw or arm. Some notice tingling sensations in the left arm. Some also notice shortness of breath, sweating or nausea. The discomfort may come on when you are not active, especially when the problem first starts. It may awaken you from sleep.

The problem is that in some cases the above typical feelings may not happen. There may be only pain in the jaw, neck or arm. The pain might be sharp instead of as described above. It may seem to be mere "indigestion." There may not be any discomfort at all (this is called "silent" coronary heart disease).

When any of the discomforts described above is caused by coronary heart disease it is called angina pectoris. The discomfort usually lasts a few minutes or less. It usually is relieved by resting or by a medication called nitroglycerin. A nitroglycerin tablet is placed under the tongue and allowed to dissolve. Many persons can predict which activity will bring on the angina pectoris in their own case and therefore avoid some episodes.

If you feel any of the above discomfort you should contact your physician. If you notice the discomfort for the first time or if it lasts longer than a few minutes then you should contact your physician immediately. If you already know that you have coronary heart disease or angina pectoris and the discomfort lasts longer than usual or comes on more often than usual you should contact your physician immediately.

The reason for the urgency if the discomfort is new or changes or lasts longer than a few minutes is the danger of an untreated heart attack (myocardial infarction). Heart attacks which happen outside the hospital may have up to 50 percent death rate. This is usually due to dangerous irregular heart rhythms which can happen in a heart attack. If these happen in a hospital they can often be treated quickly and effectively. If these happen outside the hospital, there is not good treatment and death may result.

Try not to ignore or deny these feelings if they happen. Find good medical care for proper diagnosis and treatment of this life-threatening disease. If you aren't sure how to reach a physician then go to a nearby hospital emergency room or call for emergency assistance. Some newer treatments are available for heart attacks which can only be used if the problem is detected within the first few hours. These treatments use newer medications to decrease or dissolve the blockage in the coronary artery which causes the heart attack. If successful, these newer treatments may help limit or prevent permanent damage to the heart muscle itself. This could prevent heart failure and death. These medicines are not available in all areas. Your physician can tell you if your area has these treatments available.

Don't wait to see changes before you take action. You may see rapid breathing, sweating, nausea or vomiting. But all may appear normal. If any of the above feelings happen to you then take action quickly. If you are not sure what to do, you should call your physician for advice.

Your physician will order an electrocardiogram (ECG or EKG). You may have other tests such as chest x-ray, blood tests, or exercise electrocardiogram. The most specific test to tell whether there is coronary artery disease and blockage present is coronary angiography. In this test the filling of the coronary arteries is seen directly on x-ray and a specific, accurate diagnosis can usually be made. This test is not necessary in each case. It can tell how much narrowing is present in the coronary arteries. It can tell if there has been damage to the heart muscle itself and how well the heart is working as a pump for the blood. Coronary angiography is done in the hospital using local anesthesia with rapid recovery after a few hours. There is little pain and discomfort involved. (Cardiologists and cardiac surgeons can use this test to tell the chance of success for treatments to decrease the blockage or surgery such as coronary bypass surgery.) Your physician can advise you and give you further specific details for your own situation.

Many medications are used to treat coronary heart disease. Nitroglycerin tablets are given for episodes of angina pectoris as described above. These are usually carried with a person at all times to be used when needed. Other medications are also used, depending on the individual situation. These include groups of medications called beta blockers (such as propranolol), other nitroglycerin-like products available by tablet, skin patch, and aerosol, and calcium-channel blockers (such as diltiazem, nicardipine, and verapamil).

When the chest discomfort is new or increasing in frequency or severity or when the discomfort is longer lasting and heart attack is suspected then treatment may be required in the hospital. This allows the underlying problem to be stabilized and allows proper diagnosis and treatment to begin. Each person is different. Treatment must be individualized depending on each situation.

Remember—diagnosis and treatment can't begin until the problem is recognized. Don't ignore warning signs and feelings. If you have ANY unexplained chest discomfort talk with your physician.

Other Causes of Chest Discomfort

A blood clot which lodges in an artery in the lung (pulmonary embolus) often causes chest pain. The discomfort may be hard to distinguish from the pain of coronary heart disease because it can also cause dull pain in the front of the chest. However, the pain of pulmonary embolus is often sharp and made worse by taking a breath, especially with deep inspiration. There is usually shortness of breath which can be severe. Cough may be present with blood in the sputum when coughing.

Rapid breathing is often present with shortness of breath, even with no activity. There may be sweating, rapid pulse, and fever. Blood clots may originate in the veins of the legs and pelvis. In some (but by no means all) cases there may be swelling or pain in the legs, especially in the calves. Don't wait until you see changes to seek medical care.

Tests usually include chest x-ray, measurement of oxygen levels in the blood, and lung scan. The lung scan is very important in making the diagnosis of pulmonary embolus. An x-ray of the arteries of the lungs may occasionally be needed to confirm the diagnosis.

Treatment requires medications which limit blood clot formation, heparin and warfarin (Coumadin). Heparin is most commonly used as initial treatment while in hospital and is given by vein. Other newer medications which dissolve blood clots are now available for use in some cases. Coumadin is a tablet which is taken as an outpatient after initial treatment in hospital. These medications require close supervision by your physician. Treatment of pulmonary embolus is extremely important since if left untreated it can lead to further serious illness and death.

There are other serious causes of discomfort in the chest. These include discomfort which originates in the esophagus or stomach but is felt in the chest. This can be caused by *esophagitis*, which is inflammation in the esophagus and is often made worse after eating. It can be very difficult to tell the difference between pain caused by heart disease and pain from the esophagus. "Indigestion" may be the only feeling and may be ignored as not important unless these facts are known.

Chest pain can be caused by inflammation in the wall of the chest, often just to the left of the sternum (breastbone). The problem is called *costochondritis*. This pain can be severe, sharp or dull, and is usually made worse by breathing and movement. Because the pain may be severe and is worse with breathing it can cause much anxiety. Many persons fear they are having a heart attack. Although the pain can be prominent, this cause is not serious. It is treated by applying moist heat and using medications which decrease the inflammation. These medicines are discussed on page 158.

Chest pain can also be caused by *anxiety*. The pain does not usually have the patterns as described for the above causes, but is often constant with no predictable causes or relief. It is often present in a person who shows others signs of stress and anxiety. Other causes of discomfort in the chest need to be ruled out before this diagnosis is made since anxiety is common in all of the above more serious causes of chest discomfort. Treatment includes reassurance that no other serious disease is present and management of the anxiety.

There are many other causes of discomfort and pain in the chest. Our purpose is not to list each one. Each person is different. Don't try to diagnose your own chest discomfort. Let your physician help you manage this problem so that quick, proper diagnosis and treatment can be completed. Then you can gain peace of mind knowing that the chest discomfort you have experienced is not potentially life-threatening.

■ COLD (RHINITIS)

Rhinitis is infection of the nose lining. Nasal discharge, fever, and a tired sensation (malaise) characterize it. It is usually self-limiting, but occasionally requires medication to control it. It is important to treat quickly in the elderly or in the very young, those with diabetes mellitus, or anyone with a lowered immune response or lowered ability to fight infection, such as those persons with AIDS or who are taking chemotherapy.

■ COUGH

Coughing which persists after a cold or other respiratory infection or a new cough which is persistent is considered abnormal. Some helpful points to tell your physician are how long the cough has been present; whether any activities or exposures seem to make it worse; if the cough produces sputum (phlegm) or blood; and whether you notice any other different feelings. For any persistent cough even with no other feelings you should see a physician.

The cause of the cough may cause other changes which you can see such as blood in the sputum when you cough. However, changes which you can see would be late changes for most important causes of cough. Do not wait until you notice changes if a cough is persistent. See your physician.

A discussion and examination will guide the physician in ordering tests. These may include chest x-ray and blood tests. In some cases it is necessary to see a lung specialist for further tests including bronchoscopy (direct examination of the bronchial tubes). Your physician will guide you.

Treatment depends on the cause of the cough. Medications including cough syrups may suppress the cough but the underlying cause should be found and treated.

■ DEMENTIA (See page 154.)

■ DENTAL CARE

Cavities in teeth can happen at any age. The high rate of cavities found in youth and adolescence usually fades and becomes less of a problem in adults. Mature adults usually require repair of previously restored teeth more often than new cavities. Decay in the mature adult often affects the roots of the teeth rather than the crowns. The material of roots is softer than the enamel of crowns. The gums normally gradually recede, the surfaces of the roots of the teeth are more exposed, less protected, and become much more susceptible to cavities. This requires careful brushing and care to insure cleanliness.

A toothbrush, water, irrigators, dental floss and tape, and gum stimulators all have a place in home dental care for mature adults. You should select the components that you need to give proper care. Your dentist can advise which of these you need to accomplish the job.

Try to brush each tooth surface, clean in between all teeth, and stimulate the gum tissue around each tooth once in each 24-hour period. This cleaning disrupts the plaque and bacteria that constantly form and are a natural part of the mouth. Plaque and bacteria accumulate normally regardless of eating habits or diet. Even people who are ill and not eating must still keep a clean mouth.

Select a convenient time during the day to do a thorough cleaning of the mouth. Many adults brush the last moment before going to bed. They are tired, irritable and rush to finish without thinking of the desired results.

Regardless of age, everyone can benefit from a continuous use of fluorides such as solutions in mouthwash and in toothpaste. The very small amounts of fluoride contained in these over-the-counter products help replace the lost hardness in tooth outer enamel that is removed by the action of bacteria and saliva. The safety of these fluorides is now well established. Fluorides in higher doses than normal must be obtained by prescription.

Have periodic checkups. Because everyone is different, if you are in good dental health with proper home dental care, you will need less frequent dental visits. First achieve the stability of a healthy mouth. Then your dentist can guide you to the frequency of visits needed for office dental care.

Accidents will happen. A fractured tooth or filling will periodically occur to everyone, and necessary repair must take place. Do not feel guilty or ill-treated, as even the most expensive automobile comes with a spare tire!

■ DEPRESSION

Low spirits or sadness are common feelings in normal persons. In most cases these are normal reactions to events which make us unhappy or interfere with our lives. In most of us these feelings are temporary and do not become more limiting. When these feelings of sadness, low spirits, and loss of ability to have pleasure from any part of life become severe then the problem is considered depression. Other feelings may be loss of appetite, difficulty sleeping, early morning awakening, trouble concentrating, feelings of guilt and worthlessness, feeling as if there is no hope, and even thoughts or expressions of suicide or death.

The visible signs are the overall appearance of one who is sad, feels low spirits, and hopelessness. There is usually little expression on the face. There may be loss of weight.

It is best not to wait for visible signs to appear. If there is limitation or interference in daily life, if there is persistent sadness and gloominess, and especially if there are thoughts of death or suicide then a physician should be contacted.

Discussion and examination will usually give the physician a clinical impression of depression. Tests will be planned to be sure no other medical problems are present which might contribute to or cause depression. The physician may suggest an evaluation by a psychiatrist or clinical psychologist.

Treatment includes attention to those factors in personal life which may be contributing to depression. Medications are often used and may be helpful along with visits with the psychiatrist or psychologist. In severe cases, especially when death or suicidal thoughts have been expressed, hospitalization for treatment is needed.

■ DIABETES MELLITUS

Diabetes mellitus is a medical problem in which the level of glucose in the blood is found to be abnormally high. The actual cause is not known and no cure is available. However, good medical treatment is available so that the disease is usually able to be controlled and many of its complications avoided.

The abnormal elevation in blood glucose may be found on routine examination, but most persons have begun to have feelings of fatigue, weight loss, increase in volume of urine, increased thirst, burning in the feet, changes in vision, infections, or other problems.

There may be no visible changes in appearance. Vision may change or become blurred. If the level of glucose remains elevated then complications including weight loss, severe fatigue, frequent urination of large amounts, increased thirst, more frequent infections and severe illness requiring hospital treatment may happen. Over a period of time, diabetes mellitus can cause a higher risk of kidney disease, loss of vision, higher chance of atherosclerosis with blockage of the arteries, and other medical problems.

After discussion and examination your physician will plan tests including blood tests to confirm the diagnosis of diabetes mellitus. It is important that other medical problems be evaluated which might cause the diabetes to be more difficult to control. Also, since diabetes mellitus is a risk factor for coronary heart disease (as discussed on page 48), it is important that all other risk factors be evaluated for control.

Treatment includes treatment of any other underlying problems such as infections. Diabetes mellitus may require insulin treatment to control the blood glucose. Your physician will decide if this is necessary. In this case proper use of the insulin and proper injection techniques will be needed. Close follow up to be sure that blood glucose is controlled is important. A diet will also be prescribed which will allow desirable body weight to be maintained. The diet takes into account body weight and build, daily activities and exercise and other individual needs. Diet is extremely important in controlling diabetes mellitus. A regular exercise program will be prescribed according to each person's abilities and needs.

If insulin treatment is not needed then a diet will be prescribed which will maintain body weight at desirable levels (including weight loss if overweight). The daily activity and exercise will also be taken into account. Those who perform heavy physical activity will require more calories each day. A regular exercise program will be prescribed which is safe for each person.

Your physician can guide you so that possible complications including changes in vision from eye complications can be controlled. Diabetes is a major cause of blindness in the United States. Not all diabetics develop diabetic eye disease, but the likelihood of such changes increases with the length of time that a person has diabetes. In early stages of the eye disease, the patient is not aware of any vision problem. With time, retinal blood vessels begin to leak leading to decreased vision, hemorrhage into the eye, retinal detachment, glaucoma, and possibly blindness.

With the advent of the laser, the ophthalmologist may be able to seal those leaking vessels before they have a chance to cause vision loss. All diabetics need at least yearly ophthalmologic examinations so that the condition can be diagnosed early and treated to prevent the loss of sight.

With control of blood glucose there should be improvement in fatigue and ability to carry out daily activities more easily. Control of the diabetes mellitus is needed as part of the management of risk factors to prevent coronary heart disease. Follow up with your physician is usually needed at around 3-month intervals if blood glucose remains controlled and no other problems happen. Your physician can help you decide what is best for your own situation.

■ DIZZINESS

Dizziness is a sensation of unsteadiness, or a sense of swirling around in a circle, or having objects around you appearing to move in a circle. This is very common. It can originate from the aging process, an infection, or blockage of blood vessels to the inner ear. Diseases of the nerves to the brain or the brain itself may also cause dizziness. It is not always simple to be certain of the origin of the dizziness and thus specific tests may be selected according to the symptoms. It is not necessarily an indication of a "stroke" or tumor. This symptom can be treated effectively in most cases once the source of the symptom is identified—the ear, the brain, the blood vessels or other causes. It is important to see a physician to identify the cause in order to offer appropriate therapy.

■ DRUG ABUSE

Americans abuse alcohol more than any other drug. Society's casual attitude and even endorsement of drug use through advertising encourage overprescribing practices by physicians and abuse of illegal and prescription drugs. Lessening the demand for drugs depends almost entirely on individuals making personal decisions to abstain from use and getting help when they can't stop on their own. Personal abstinence broadcasts the commitment that drugs do not provide an acceptable alternative to the solution of life's problems.

The chemical structure and action on the mind varies tremendously from drug to drug, but drugs fall into several major groups. Sedatives include alcohol and other depressant drugs. They slow all mental processes. Death results from overdose by slowing the respiratory rate. In contrast, stimulants act on the brain in the opposite way. Cocaine is the most widely abused of this group. Cocaine is easily modified into "Crack" which can be inhaled by smoking it. This chemical change allows free base cocaine to reach the brain, heart, and other organs in very high concentrations. Several famous individuals, frequently athletes, have died after using drugs in this way.

Narcotics anesthetize the brain by a different action than sedatives do. Many narcotic addicts, particularly among more mature adults, are created unintentionally while being treated with prescription narcotics for pain.

Many complications occur from the use of drugs. AIDS and hepatitis are transmitted by contaminated needles used for intravenous drug administration. Almost all abused drugs can cause birth defects, and almost every organ in the body may be damaged by the use of drugs. Unfortunately a most devastating effect may occur in weakening a society which depends on clear mental functioning for survival.

Any use of illicit drugs should be considered addiction. All the principles of denial, dependence, and addiction described previously for alcohol also apply to other drugs. Like alcoholism, drug addiction treatment depends heavily on mutual help groups such as Narcotics Anonymous and Cocaine Anonymous. Medical treatment must sometimes be sought since withdrawal can be difficult and prolonged. Drug use produces an altered mental status that can lead to unpredictable, violent, or self-destructive behavior. The compulsion to use drugs can continue long after the person has stopped using, so maintaining contact with a support group is essential.

Fortunately recovery from alcohol and drug problems restores most of the damage the addiction produced. Sober alcoholics and drug addicts have no more emotional problems than the normal population. The struggle to overcome an addiction frequently prepares the addict to handle everyday problems of life more constructively than ever. Recovery from substance abuse problems requires an individual to live in a way that drugs are not necessary to endure whatever life brings.

Your physician can give you advice if you or someone you know needs treatment for drug abuse.

■ DRY EYES

Eye dryness is a common malady that results from aging effects on the lacrimal glands which produce the tears. This may be relieved by the use of artificial tears which can be bought over the counter. If no relief from the artificial tears occurs, then a visit to your physician is suggested.

■ DRYNESS OF THE MOUTH

A lack of saliva may cause dryness in the mouth, difficulty chewing and swallowing, and an increase in dental cavities. Saliva produced is a lubricant, containing many chemicals that bathe the teeth, protecting them from acid-producing bacteria. Dry mouth can be a side effect of antihistamines or other medications. There is no excellent treatment available. Rinsing the mouth frequently with water, the use of special oral rinses, toothpastes, and chewing gum may give some improvement. Severe dryness in the mouth should be managed with the help of a dentist and a physician.

■ EAR NOISE (TINNITUS)

Noise such as ringing in the ear is called *tinnitus*. This problem may affect up to 36 million adults in the United States. The sound may be ringing, roaring like a sea shell, or like that of steam escaping. It may last from several seconds to all of our waking hours. There may be a pulsating component of the noise which is due to transmitted blood impulses within the blood vessels in the ear. Continuous tinnitus may also have hearing loss or dizziness along with it. It is important to realize that this is a common problem. Usually this is only an annoyance but it can be the sign of more serious problems and should be evaluated. A previous history of noise exposure with hearing loss is common along with the tinnitus. Tinnitus is often more troubling when the other noise levels are low such as at bedtime. Sometimes using a radio or television at low levels will cover the annoying tinnitus and allow sleep. A visit to an ENT physician may be helpful. The tinnitus may not be able to be completely eliminated, but it is important to rule out other underlying disease which may cause the tinnitus.

■ EPISTAXIS (NOSEBLEED)

Epistaxis is a nosebleed which can occur at any age. It may be due to rhinitis, as in a cold or where there is a reduction in environmental humidity (air conditioning or heating, either central or a fireplace). The immediate treatment is to hold the head forward in a bent over position and apply an ice bag to both forehead and the back of the neck. Holding the soft part of the nose and pinching it together is helpful. Aspirin and other medications may increase the chances of bleeding. If bleeding does not stop in 15 minutes by holding the nose and sitting appropriately, then contact your family physician or an ENT physician. The bleeding can at times be related to hypertension or to other significant diseases.

■ EYE DISORDERS

There are several conditions which are not normal aging changes in the eye. These conditions can lead to severe permanent vision loss and/or pain. While it is important to recognize the early symptoms and signs of these conditions, it is a fact that sometimes there are no warning signs. The best way to prevent the loss of sight is to have periodic eye examinations by an ophthalmologist. For the average healthy adult over age 40, a complete eye examination should be performed routinely every two years. If a specific medical problem is found, the need for a complete eye exam may be more frequent.

Eye and Vison Warning Signs. The warning signs which should alert one to seek attention by an ophthalmologist are:

1. Sudden onset of new floaters or change in pattern of floaters (contact immediately)
2. Any eye pain (contact immediately)
3. Waviness of vision (contact immediately)
4. Temporary vision loss or the onset of a blind spot (contact immediately)
5. Decreased vision which cannot be corrected with glasses
6. Scratchy, burning, red eyes for more than one week
7. Any medical condition such as diabetes for which a physician recommends referral

Preventive eye care may permit early detection of visual problems associated with aging that might otherwise lead to severe permanent visual loss.

Glaucoma. Many elderly people are affected by glaucoma and do not even know it. There are usually no early symptoms and most patients are not aware of anything being wrong.

Glaucoma, in most cases, is elevated pressure inside of the eye. This increase in pressure causes damage to the optic nerve and therefore leads to vision loss. Most of the time the disease progresses slowly. Usually there is no pain. Sometimes, in susceptible people, the pressure rises rapidly and the patient experiences sudden decreased vision and intense eye pain. In either case, loss of vision from glaucoma can usually be prevented if the disease is detected and treated early.

When glaucoma is suspected, a test which can detect subtle vision loss called a visual field test may be ordered. If the ophthalmologist feels that glaucoma is present, the pressure can usually be lowered with eye drops or pills. In rare cases, laser surgery or an operative procedure is necessary to lower the pressure and preserve sight.

■ FACIAL WRINKLES

Wrinkles are common to all of us with aging. Besides having chosen no wrinkle genes from our parents, our choices are limited. For fine wrinkles around the lower lids, cheeks, and some about the lips, the new cream Retin-A is of benefit. This is not without its deleterious effects and thus your physician, facial plastic surgeon, or dermatologist should be seen. For the deeper wrinkles and aging folds, an operation (facelift, rhytidectomy) designed for your particular needs can be done. A facial plastic otolaryngologist or general plastic surgeon should be consulted for this therapy.

■ FACIAL PAIN

Facial pain may be mild or very intense and usually occurs in the cheek or in the forehead region on one side of the face. It can be continuous or simply a stabbing, intermittent pain. The pain may be slow or rapid in onset and it may feel dull or very sharp. It may occur only occasionally or several times every day. It may last for only a few seconds or it may last an hour. This pain may come from the teeth or sinus or there may be no clear origin. It may come after pressure on the skin, tooth or sinus or may require no contact to initiate it. Evaluation by an internist, an ENT physician, or a neurologist is in order. Treatment usually requires medication and depending on its cause, rarely an operation is needed.

■ FAINTING (SYNCOPE)

Sudden temporary loss of consciousness may be preceded by weakness, dizziness, or lightheadedness. Or, there may be no warning feelings at all. The concern is that some causes may be serious including irregular heart rhythms which cause a decrease in blood flow to the brain. Especially when it happens for the first time, an episode of syncope (the medical term for sudden temporary loss of consciousness) needs immediate medical attention.

Your physician can guide you as to which tests are needed to be sure no serious underlying disease is present.

■ FATIGUE

Fatigue is common with physical or emotional stress. It becomes abnormal when we feel exhaustion or tiredness out of proportion to what we would usually expect from our schedule of rest and activity. Fatigue can be a sign of other medical problems as well as emotional or mental health problems. You may have no other feelings or symptoms. Or you may have other feelings from the underlying problem. If you feel fatigue which you cannot easily explain by your schedule of rest, activity and diet then you should see your physician.

Because there are so many possible causes of abnormal fatigue, most important would be a discussion with your physician and a physical examination. Then guided by these results, some specific tests can be ordered to avoid a multitude of tests.

Treatment depends entirely on the cause of the fatigue. Once a specific cause is found, treatment can be planned.

■ FEVER

Our body's temperature is normally 98.6 degrees F. or 37 degrees C. If it is noticed that body temperature is above normal levels for more than a few days then you should contact your physician. The most common problem is an acute infection. Fever is common with respiratory infections and viral infections and usually disappears as other signs of the infection go away. If fever persists after other signs of infection have disappeared then it is reasonable to ask your physician for advice.

If fever appears with no other signs and lasts more than a few days then further evaluation is needed. There are many different causes of persistent fever. If it is not clear from discussion and examination then a number of studies may be needed to be sure no other diseases are present. As in other problems, the better the information which is available to your physician the more efficient the investigation will be—and the fewer the number of tests that may be required to find the underlying cause.

■ FIBROSITIS

A common cause of pain in muscles and joints of the arms, legs, neck, and back is fibrositis. It is one of the most common causes of pain and stiffness. It is most common in females. Five times as many females are affected as males. The cause is unknown, although some cases have begun following injury which may be quite mild or even emotional in nature. Some researchers feel there may be a viral cause. Some think it may also involve a disorder of sleep. The term fibrositis implies that there is inflammation of fibrous tissue in the muscles and other tissues, but this has not been proven when samples of those tissues were studied. This problem goes by other names including fibromyalgia, fibromyositis, and tension myalgias.

Most persons feel widespread aching in their muscles and joints. The areas most commonly affected are the neck, shoulders, elbows, knees and back. Although there may be difficulty doing daily work or caring for the home, most persons can complete these duties despite not feeling well. The symptoms and feelings usually come and go and commonly are associated with fatigue, headache, and depression. Many persons describe difficulty sleeping. They may be unable to go to sleep or may not feel rested when they awaken in the morning.

There is no joint swelling, no loss of movement of the joints, and no true muscle weakness. Usually the only abnormal findings are tender areas (trigger points) over the neck, shoulder blades, lower back, elbows, and knees. In fact, if a joint is warm or swollen or does not move properly then there is probably a different problem present. Fibrositis can happen alone. The diseases that may be associated with fibrositis are other kinds of arthritis such as systemic lupus erythematosus (SLE or lupus), rheumatoid arthritis, polymyositis, polymyalgia rheumatica, and other internal organ diseases.

The diagnosis is difficult as there are no specific laboratory studies, and no abnormal x-ray findings are present from fibrositis. There may be a need to have more than one examination to be sure no other disorders are being overlooked.

Fibrositis may be a chronic illness and the various treatments may not always be successful. Most specialists advise modest exercise with or without physical therapy, biofeedback to learn muscle relaxation, and avoidance of stress if that is a contributor. Nonsteroidal antiinflammatory drugs, medication to help gain more restful sleep, and local injection of trigger points may be helpful in the treatment of fibrositis. Although there is research in progress now, no obvious breakthroughs are on the near horizon.

■ FLOATERS

People of all ages are often disturbed by floaters. They appear as specks seen especially when looking at a light background. They literally "float" in and out of view. As one gets older, it is highly likely that these floaters will increase due to the changes in the clear gel-like fluid called vitreous which fills the eye. Most floaters are not associated with serious eye disease, however, a sudden increase in the number of floaters may signal a torn or detached retina. A broken blood vessel in the eye can also produce a sudden increase in floaters with subsequent decreased vision. It is always wise to see an ophthalmologist to determine if floaters are harmless or the beginning of a more serious problem.

■ GLAUCOMA (See page 184)

■ GOUT

Gout is a form of arthritis that may cause sudden onset of severe pain. The pain in an acute attack of gout becomes progressively worse over a few hours. The large toe is the most commonly involved joint and is the first joint attacked in 75 percent of cases of gout. The joint is usually swollen, warm, tender to touch and may be red. Occasionally more than one joint may be attacked at one time.

Diagnosis is made most accurately by examining a sample of fluid obtained from the joint. Under the microscope, crystals are seen which confirm gout. A blood test may be taken to measure the level of uric acid. If elevated, this makes a person more likely to develop gout, although it alone does not make the diagnosis definite.

Treatment of the acute attack of gout uses medications including indomethacin, colchicine or others. Relief usually comes within a few days but the entire attack may last longer. Deposits of uric acid may collect in the kidneys and form kidney stones. Medications are available which can help prevent future attacks of gout and treat this type of kidney stone. Your physician can guide you in the use of these medications depending on your individual situation.

■ GUM DISEASE

Diseases of the gums can be acute or may be long-lasting. Infection of the gums is the most common of these ailments in mature adults. Proper diagnosis and supervision by the dentist can allow a person to help manage much of this problem just as other areas of health are managed.

Acute abscess in the gum can be caused by infection in a pocket or crevice near a tooth. The pain and swelling can be intense, similar to a toothache. Chronic gum infection usually includes bleeding when teeth are brushed and frequent halitosis but may not be painful.

This can accompany bone loss around the teeth and may promote tooth loss.

■ GYNECOLOGICAL CONCERNS

Pelvic infections are common in mature women. There may be no symptoms at all or there may be pain in the pelvis, fever, and chills. These infections are usually sexually transmitted. After discussion and examination a diagnosis is often made after examination of a specimen from the vagina or cervix. The most common causes are chlamydia and gonorrhea. It is important that antibiotic treatment is started early and the course of treatment completed to completely eradicate the infection. The sexual partner may need treatment in many cases. Your physician can give you specific suggestions.

Infections of the vagina (vaginitis) are common in mature adults. The most common cause of such infections in the vagina and the adjacent external areas is Candida (yeast).

Candida (yeast) is commonly present in the vaginal area. Infection happens when there is an overgrowth of the Candida organisms. There may be itching in the vaginal area. There may be a discharge from the vagina, often thick, white and curd-like. The diagnosis may be made by the physician's examination. Several treatments are available including creams and suppositories. The male sexual partner does not usually require separate treatment.

Trichomonas infection is usually sexually transmitted. The infection is present in the vagina and also in the glands at the opening of the vagina. There is usually a foul-smelling yellow vaginal discharge. At times there may be no symptoms. Metronidazole is the treatment of choice and is given to the sexual partner as well to eradicate the infection.

Genital herpes infections are referred to as Type I or Type II. Type II is most common. When first infected there may be fever, chills, with pain and swelling around the opening of the vagina. There may be problems in urination. It is usually sexually transmitted. The incubation period (the time from first exposure to signs of disease) is usually three weeks or less.

Diagnosis of herpes infection is made by the physician. Treatment includes local care of the skin, fluids, pain medications, and acyclovir which is a medication directed against the herpes virus.

Gonorrhea is sexually transmitted and in women may not cause symptoms until a severe infection has occurred. With infection of the vagina there may be a thick discharge. With more severe infection there may also be fever, chills, and pain in the abdomen and pelvis. The diagnosis is made by the physician by examination and with other tests including cultures. Treatment depends on the severity of the infection and individual situation—antibiotics such as penicillins, tetracyclines and others are used. If not treated the infection may cause an abscess in the Fallopian tubes and pelvis. This can also lead to chronic pelvic pain and infertility.

Syphilis is a sexually transmitted disease which is most commonly noticed as a painless sore outside the vagina. If this is not treated, progression of syphilis may occur even though the sore may disappear. Problems from syphilis may appear weeks or months later as rash and other problems. Years later there may be permanent damage to the heart, brain and other organs if untreated. Diagnosis is made by examination of the initial sore and by blood tests. Treatment is with penicillin or other appropriate antibiotics.

Menopause

Menopause refers to a woman's final menstrual period. This happens in the period of life between a woman's reproductive stage and her non-reproductive stage. This period of life is referred to as the climacteric. The average age of menopause is around 51 years. Most women have menopause between ages 45 and 55.

After age 35 there is a gradual decrease to low levels of the female estrogen hormones. This is due to lower production of estrogens by the ovaries. Several changes happen at this time, probably mainly as a result of the change in estrogen levels. About 85 percent of women have hot flushes around the time of menopause. These are sudden hot sensations often in the neck, upper body or throughout the body. There is often flushing of the skin and sweating. There may be shivering, nausea, and palpitations. The episode usually lasts a few minutes. These may happen during the day but often happen at night and interrupt sleep. The interruption of sleep may lead to increase in irritability, fatigue, and daytime sleepiness. Usually these symptoms last less than 2 years, but some persons have them for 5 years or longer.

Other feelings include headache, anxiety, feeling inadequate, and decrease in concentration. Dryness of the skin and membranes can result in dryness of the vagina with discharge and with painful intercourse. There may be frequency of urination with a feeling of urgency to empty the bladder. Osteoporosis (thinning of the bones) may progress more rapidly during this period.

Some of the problems of this period of life may be affected by a woman's understanding of these symptoms. Many symptoms may suggest that some other disease is present. The fatigue and irritability may make it more difficult for family members to understand. Support and understanding from family and friends can make this time much easier.

Tests are available to be sure no other medical problems are present. Treatment is also available in the form of estrogen replacement. Estrogen treatment improves and often controls the hot flushes, dryness in the vagina and urinary symptoms. It also is a major part of controlling the risk of osteoporosis which happens when estrogen levels decrease at the time of menopause. The lack of estrogens is the most common cause of osteoporosis in women after menopause.

There are some possible side effects of estrogen treatment. Estrogen treatment is not recommended for all women. Talk with your physician or gynecologist and decide what choice is best in your own situation.

Cancer Tests

Pap Smear (Papanicolaou Smear). A test which is performed in the office and is very effective in detecting cervical cancer and precancer. It is a painless and inexpensive way to control this cancer. It is recommended that women have a pap smear test performed once a year (or other schedule if recommended by your physician or gynecologist).

Endometrial Biopsy. A simple test used to evaluate the lining of the womb (uterus). This test is used to further diagnose problems including heavy bleeding from the vagina. It may be a part of the evaluation of fertility and other problems.

Dilatation and Curettage (D and C). An outpatient procedure in which the mouth of the womb (uterus) is dilated and the lining of the uterus is scraped. This allows a sample to be examined under a microscope for abnormalities. This procedure is most commonly performed after age 30. This may be performed as part of the diagnosis and treatment of abnormal bleeding from the vagina.

Laparoscopy. Laparoscopy uses an endoscope which transmits light back to the viewer and allows direct examination of many of the internal organs. This is done through a small incision through the umbilicus in the lower abdomen. The pelvic organs including the ovaries, Fallopian tubes, appendix, and uterus can be evaluated in this manner. It is an outpatient procedure which may allow other treatments including tubal ligation (interruption of the Fallopian tubes to prevent further pregnancy). This direct examination may also help in the evaluation of other problems. The use of this test depends on the individual situation.

Breast Self-Examination. Women can help control the most common kind of cancer by regular self-examination of the breasts and with the use of a type of x-ray of the breasts called mammogram. When used together, researchers have shown that this is a very effective way to detect cancers in the breasts. If these cancers are found early the treatment is effective and much more likely to result in a cure. Self-examination and mammogram are easy to do, painless and safe.

Women should examine their own breasts about once each month. A good time to choose is following the menstrual cycle. After menopause or after hysterectomy then choose a regular time each month for this self-exam. A convenient time is often after bathing or before retiring at night. Looking in a mirror, compare the breasts to see if there are any differences in appearance. There is often a slight difference in size of breasts which is considered normal. Check to see if there is a difference in the breasts from swelling, changes in the skin, or changes in the nipples. Check to see if there is any discharge from the nipples or any difference in appearance of the nipples.

Then, by gentle palpation starting at the nipple each breast is examined. An easy way is to examine the breasts one-fourth at a time. While lying supine the breast tissue is firmly pressed against the chest wall. Check for any lumps, firmness, or changes in consistency of the breast tissue. Remember that there is normally breast tissue present which is made of glands and fatty tissue. Any changes from month to month will be noticeable. Any new lump, firmness, discharge from the nipple or other new feeling on examination is important. If any change is present then you should contact your physician.

After a few months most women can know quite well what is "normal" in their own examination. The longer this monthly examination is continued, the easier it will be to notice subtle differences and early problems. Combined with physician examination of the breasts at regular intervals and mammogram, women can know that a most effective early detection system is in place. This is an important part of the plan for early detection of cancer—when treatment is most effective.

Mammogram. An x-ray which can detect breast abnormalities before they are able to be felt by examination. It is painless, effective, and requires a small and acceptable amount of radiation from the examination. Newer techniques now use a lower amount of radiation. A mammogram can detect most breast cancers, often before they are otherwise noticeable. Combined with self-examination and regular physician examination it is the most effective way to detect breast cancer early.

Researchers recommend regular mammograms although there are some differences in specific times for the examination. Your physician can guide you in your own situation.

Hysterectomy. Hysterectomy refers to removal of the uterus by surgery. There are specific problems which may require hysterectomy. The most common are cancer, endometriosis, fibroid tumors of the uterus, and as a last resort in bleeding which is not able to be controlled by medications or other treatment.

In total hysterectomy the entire uterus and cervix are removed. In subtotal hysterectomy the cervix is not removed. If the ovaries and Fallopian tubes are also removed it is referred to as hysterectomy and salpingo-oophorectomy. When possible the ovaries are not removed, depending on the individual situation. Some of the factors taken into account are the medical problem, age, and good medical judgment. Usually it is preferred when possible *not* to remove the ovaries before age 40. After hysterectomy, there are no menstrual periods or pregnancy. Following hysterectomy sexual function is usually unchanged but may be enhanced if the previous problem was limiting sexual function.

If the ovaries are removed before the age of menopause then estrogen replacement treatment may be used. This usually avoids some of the problems caused by lack of the estrogen normally produced by the ovaries including dryness and shrinkage of tissue in the vagina.

Be sure that you understand the need for treatments which include hysterectomy. You should know the advantages and risks and what the alternative treatment might be. Then with your physician you can decide what the best choice is for your own situation.

Fibroid Tumor of the Uterus (Leiomyoma). Fibroid tumors of the uterus are very common benign tumors. About 20–25 percent of women eventually have fibroid tumors of the uterus. There may be no feelings or signs. There may be abnormal bleeding from the vagina.

In many cases no specific treatment is needed. In certain situations it is possible that surgery might be needed. These include suspicion of cancer, rapidly enlarging tumors, uncontrolled bleeding, or problems with fertility. These assessments and decisions are usually made over a period of time by your physician.

Vaginal Bleeding (Bleeding from the Vagina). Abnormal vaginal bleeding is a common problem with many different causes. Many causes are not serious, but the bleeding may be the only sign of a serious underlying medical problem. Any change from the usual menstrual pattern should be discussed with your physician. This includes heavier than usual bleeding, longer or more frequent menstrual periods, bleeding between periods or vaginal bleeding after menopause. No other feelings or signs need to be present to suggest the need to contact your physician.

Some of the most common causes of abnormal vaginal bleeding in mature adults are irregular shedding of the lining of the uterus, fibroid tumors of the uterus, infections, pregnancy, and tumors. Tumors may be benign or malignant.

Treatment depends on the cause of the bleeding. After discussion and examination your physician can give further specific suggestions for treatment.

Ovarian Cysts and Tumors. Ovarian cysts or tumors may be benign or malignant. There may be no feelings or signs and the problem may be detected on routine examination. There may be pain, the feeling of pressure in the pelvis, or change in menstrual periods. Many benign cysts resolve with medical treatment while some eventually require surgery.

Tests which may be planned after discussion and examination include sonogram of the pelvis. The sonogram is a very effective way to examine the ovaries. It is used to determine the size and other characteristics of ovaries and cysts. It is painless and requires no radiation. It is especially helpful in obese patients or if pain prevents thorough pelvic examination.

The results of the sonogram help guide treatment. Some factors which physicians use to decide whether surgery might be needed are size of the cyst, how long it has been present, the age of the patient, and whether a portion of the cyst is solid or not. These and other factors will decide whether the cyst can be followed carefully or whether there is a high enough risk of cancer to require surgery. For example, if the cyst is becoming smaller in a person of child-bearing age then the chances of cancer may be lower. On the other hand, in some persons, especially after child-bearing age, the finding of a cyst or tumor of the ovary can be the first sign of cancer in the ovary.

■ HAIR LOSS

Hair loss may be due to inherited causes, stress, and injury to the hair such as twisting, tugging, braiding, or tight rollers. Usually the hair will tolerate daily shampoo without excessive dryness. In fact, for dandruff or seborrhea it is often important to shampoo daily. Hair loss is not usually due to daily shampoo.

Other causes include infections of the scalp, internal organ diseases, hormonal changes such as menopause, and after pregnancy. Usually hair loss from one of these problems can be restored if the underlying problem is corrected.

If you notice unusual hair loss then you should ask your physician for advice.

■ HEADACHE

Headache is one of the most common medical problems. Up to 80 percent of persons may suffer from headaches at some time each year. Headaches may be mild or severe and short or long lasting. Headaches may be caused by another medical problem or may happen alone. A mild headache may be able to be ignored, while severe headaches may be totally incapacitating. For most persons there are two main concerns about headaches. One is how to relieve the pain, and the other is whether there is a serious cause of the headache.

Headaches are difficult to treat unless a specific cause is found. Therefore, pain relief may depend on finding the cause of the headache. Headaches which are mild, happen occasionally and have not changed for many years usually do not need any further tests or specific treatment. Some headaches do need further evaluation because they may be caused by another serious medical problem.

If the headache is severe or comes on suddenly, especially if headaches are not usually a problem, you should contact your physician. If there is sleepiness, weakness or numbness, or loss of consciousness with the headache you should contact your physician immediately. A headache which is "the worst headache in my life" is usually taken very seriously by a physician. If any of these signs—sudden onset, severe (especially if it is the worst ever) or if other problems are present also—then medical evaluation is needed as soon as possible.

Headaches may come on gradually and may be present for months or years. If the headache persists, becomes more frequent, more severe, or limits your activity then you should contact your physician.

A discussion with your physician may give the most important clues to the cause of the headache. The better you describe the headache, the more clues will be available. After an examination then tests may be planned including blood tests, x-rays including CT (computed tomography) scan of the head and other studies depending on your situation. Of those who complain of headache a majority do NOT turn out to have brain tumor, hypertension or other "well-known" causes of headache.

Tension headaches (muscle contraction headaches) are most common. These are more common in women than men with pain commonly felt in the front or the back of the head or in both places. Vascular headaches are also more common in women. They are felt as throbbing pain and are often felt on one side of the head. Other family members may have been affected by similar headaches. Some persons find that foods such as chocolate, cheese, or red wine may seem to trigger a headache. Cluster headaches are more common in men, especially in mature adults. These headaches are severe and often "cluster" together in attacks over weeks with long periods between attacks.

Unless a specific cause is found then treatment is difficult. This can lead to frustration in patients and physicians. Medications, exercises for the muscles of the neck, stress management and treatment of the underlying medical problems are used to give control but may not totally eliminate the headaches.

■ HEARING LOSS

Hearing loss is one of the most common physical problems as we mature and is especially common after age 65. The loss of hearing is due to degeneration of the nerve tissue in the ear. The medical term for this is presbycusis.

There may be difficulty in hearing sound levels, difficulty in understanding words, difficulty in determining the direction of a sound, or a combination of these problems. This does not mean you are "going deaf." Most frequently the loss stabilizes rather than continuing to worsen. It is important that social function and participation in activities continue. There is no specific medication or surgery which is excellent for relief, but a trial of simple hearing aids should be considered in many cases. A visit to a physician who specializes in ear disease (otolaryngologist or ear, nose and throat specialist) is important before a hearing aid is purchased. It is important to realize that this is only to aid the remaining hearing and there will be limitations which must be recognized and understood.

One cause of hearing loss which can be operated on with immediate improvement is otosclerosis. This usually has its onset early in life (age 20s and 30s). However, it may not manifest itself until after age 50. Hearing loss can be sudden in its onset at any age. This loss is of unknown cause, but can be associated with a virus, blockage of a blood vessel, or reaction to medication. This should be seen soon by an ENT physician to properly diagnose and treat this loss. Rarely, a tumor may be a cause of hearing loss.

▪ HEART FAILURE

Heart failure can begin suddenly (acute heart failure) or may come on gradually (chronic heart failure). In acute heart failure there may be sudden shortness of breath, severe weakness, the need to sit up to breathe, pain in the chest, and chest congestion with much bubbly sputum on coughing. This can happen in a person who was previously well or in someone who already has heart disease. It is an emergency and requires immediate medical care. Among the most common causes are heart attack (myocardial infarction) from coronary heart disease and hypertension. There are many other causes which can be discovered and treated after the initial emergency treatment.

Heart failure can come on gradually with slowly increasing shortness of breath, especially with activity and exertion. The shortness of breath may become worse when lying supine. Many persons find it easier to breathe in bed if more than one pillow is used to raise their head. Some may awaken at night feeling short of breath with improvement after getting up to "get some air." Swelling from excess fluid (edema) in the legs may become gradually worse and may extend to swelling in the abdomen. Weakness, nausea, and other feelings may be present. Cough, rapid breathing and bluish discoloration (cyanosis) of the hands, feet and lips may happen.

There are many causes of chronic heart failure. Your physician will plan tests including chest x-ray, electrocardiogram, blood tests, and other studies to determine the cause. Some underlying causes are specifically treatable. Some causes cannot be treated specifically but respond to the treatment of heart failure with medications including diuretics to remove excess fluid and other medications which improve the effectiveness of the pumping action of the heart. Some causes of heart failure may be corrected or improved with surgery. If other treatments fail then treatment with heart transplantation is available in some areas.

◼ HOARSENESS

Hoarseness is a common finding and indicates some abnormality in the voice box or larynx. Its cause is voice overuse, viral or bacterial infection, irritation from smoking or toxic fume inhalation, or possibly a tumor (benign or malignant). Arthritis or damage to the nerve to the larynx may cause hoarseness. Initially, you should avoid voice use for two to three days to see if the hoarseness improves. Remember that tobacco smoke is a significant larynx irritant. It is reasonable to see your ENT physician for any hoarseness lasting over 14 days.

◼ HYPOGLYCEMIA

Hypoglycemia refers to a low glucose level in the blood. When the blood glucose decreases to below about 45 mg/dl then symptoms may include sweating, nervousness, weakness, headache, and rapid heart rate. If the glucose level continues to decrease then confusion, severe weakness, seizures, and unconsciousness may result.

The diagnosis is made when the blood glucose is found to be low at the same time the above symptoms happen. Hypoglycemia is sometimes diagnosed after a test called the glucose tolerance test. This test measures the level of glucose hourly for 3–5 hours after drinking a standard amount of glucose. If none of the above feelings or symptoms happen during this test then hypoglycemia is not very likely. Some experts feel this test should not be used to make this diagnosis. Others feel that if the symptoms and feelings are reproduced during the test and the blood glucose is less than 45 mg/dl then reactive hypoglycemia may be present. Treatment includes a diet to prevent hypoglycemia with fewer carbohydrates and more protein.

Many physicians see patients who have the problem of sudden onset of weakness, sweating, palpitations, headache, and nervousness. Some of these persons do not have the same feelings during a glucose tolerance test as described above. If no other medical problems are present then some persons respond to a hypoglycemic diet. Whether this represents true hypoglycemia in each case is not known, but there may be control of the symptoms with the diet.

Hypoglycemia may also happen after fasting with low levels of blood glucose usually measured in the morning after fasting during the night. Specific medical problems can cause this form of hypoglycemia which may be dangerous.

Your physician can guide you in deciding which tests are needed when considering the diagnosis of hypoglycemia. Then treatment can be planned depending on the underlying cause.

■ INCONTINENCE AND BLADDER CONTROL

Leakage of the urine is inconvenient, but otherwise alone this leaking is not usually damaging. The underlying problem that causes the leakage can signal a situation which may lead to much more serious disease if not treated.

Stress incontinence refers to the leakage of a small amount of urine when a person coughs or strains with physical activity. This is common in women who have a "dropped bladder" (cystocele). It is also present in some men when there is weakness of one of the muscles which controls the urine flow from the bladder.

Other causes of loss of control of the urine include irritability of the bladder with spasms or contractions which may force the urine out of the bladder. This can happen during infection of the bladder. Some other diseases may cause damage to the nerve supply to the bladder. This may happen in persons with multiple sclerosis, stroke, and other diseases.

Another cause of leakage of urine from the bladder is actually due to blockage of the usual urine flow. As the pressure builds up due to the blockage, there eventually is enough pressure to force some urine out of the bladder. This would be like a dam which blocks the usual flow of water in a stream. The result is a lake with a large capacity for storage of water, but at times water spills over the dam in small amounts.

Most persons with urinary incontinence have controllable or reversible causes. This is a problem which requires thorough evaluation by your physician and urologist.

■ INSOMNIA—DIFFICULTY SLEEPING AND DAYTIME SLEEPINESS

Many persons experience difficulty with sleep at night. Often there is a night or two of sleeplessness which is related to stress in our daily lives. Usually this is temporary and disappears without further concern. Certain problems may happen to cause more serious disturbances of sleep. Two of the most common problems in older adults are problems in breathing patterns and muscle movements, especially in the legs.

Breathing changes during sleep include pauses in breathing or a reduction in air flow in breathing during sleep. Both of these events may cause a short period of partial awakening. This interruption of sleep disturbs the sleep pattern and may occur many times (up to hundreds!) each night. As many as 30–40 percent of older persons may have changes in breathing pattern during sleep even if they have no complaints. The more frequent the interruption, the more likely daytime drowsiness seems to be.

Movements of the legs may happen during sleep. These often involve slow movements of the foot or legs. These movements may cause a brief lightening or awakening from sleep just as the breathing changes above. This may disturb the sleep pattern and cause more daytime sleepiness. For example, a person who has 6 hours of uninterrupted sleep may have less daytime sleepiness than a person who has 8 or more hours of interrupted sleep.

Older persons are more likely to have problems which interrupt sleep. This contributes to more daytime sleepiness and to the belief that older people are sleepier during the day than younger people!

Problems in the length or quality of sleep can also be caused by other medical problems. There may also be an underlying sleep disorder which may be corrected. Changes in alertness during the day with excessive sleepiness should not be considered simply due to the normal process of maturity and aging. If you feel excessive daytime sleepiness or if you are not satisfied with the quality of your sleep at night there may be an underlying problem which can be corrected. Discuss this with your physician. It may be useful to see a physician who specializes in treating disorders of sleep.

■ JAW PAIN

Changes in the jaw joint are common in the aging process and are manifested by pain and tenderness in front of the ear along with clicking sounds with chewing. A history of recent dental work, gum chewing, grinding of the teeth, clenching of the jaws, or poor fitting dentures may be underlying these symptoms. Local heat application, soft diet without chewing, grinding or clenching, may be helpful. If there is no relief, then a visit to the dentist for bite analysis is beneficial.

This jaw pain may also be part of a problem including headaches and neck pain. This is called Temporomandibular Joint Syndrome

(TMJ syndrome). There are other causes of jaw pain which can be discovered by your physician and dentist.

■ JOINT PAINS (See Arthritis, page 157.)

■ KIDNEY STONES

Stones can form in the kidney, bladder or in one of the ureters (the tubes that connect the kidneys to the bladder). There may be no unusual symptoms or feelings even with large stones present. Or, there may be pain so severe that hospitalization and narcotic treatment is needed. The only sign may be small amounts of blood detectable in the urine. Or, there may be infection or blockage of the flow of urine caused by the stone with fever and severe illness.

When pain is caused by a stone in the kidney or ureter the pain is usually in the back or the side (flank). The pain is most commonly moderate to severe and is usually constant. It is often difficult to find any comfortable position.

There may be fever along with the pain if there is an infection along with the stone. The urine may appear darker or reddened due to blood.

Tests which may be ordered include IVP (intravenous pyelogram) which is an x-ray study of the kidneys, ureters, and bladder. Other tests may be needed to determine the exact location of the stone.

Once the location of the stone is known then a decision can be made for treatment plans. This may include observation to see if the stone passes. Or, it may be necessary to consider surgical treatment.

About 85 percent of all stones may pass without the need for surgery. Several types of surgery are possible if necessary. Many stones stop near the end of the ureter just before entering the bladder.

Techniques known as stone basket or stone manipulation can remove many of these stones. 60 to 75 percent of stones that require surgery can be managed using one of these methods.

Surgery for stones has become less common recently since the development of a new treatment which crushes or pulverizes stones without surgery. An energy source is used to break up the stones so that the smaller stones may pass more easily. This technique is called extracorporeal shock wave lithotripsy (ESWL). Unfortunately, this treatment is not suitable for every patient.

In some cases, the most effective form of treatment remains the older surgery in which the stone is removed from the kidney by operation.

Once the stone is removed or passed, it may be analyzed to determine the cause of the stone. Other blood and urine tests may be planned. If a specific cause of the stone is discovered, then treatment may be possible to prevent future stones and limit the growth of any remaining stones.

■ LEG PAIN

There are many different causes of pain in the legs. This discussion is not intended to be complete but will review some of the most important feelings and signs of a few common causes of leg pain. This cannot replace proper diagnosis and treatment by your physician. If you have pain in the legs which has no apparent cause or is persistent, ask your physician for advice.

Leg Pain Due to Arthritis and Bursitis

Pain in the leg can be caused by arthritis and related diseases. (See the discussion of arthritis on page 157.) Arthritis results from inflammation in or around the joints. There are many different types of arthritis. The pain may begin suddenly or gradually, often depending on the type of arthritis. The pain is usually in or near the joints of the foot, knee, or hip. Arthritis in the lower back (lumbar spine and other joints) can also cause pain in the leg.

The pain of arthritis affecting the foot, ankle, knee, or hip can be sharp or dull or may be aching with stiffness. It usually is made worse with standing or walking and may be constant. Movement of the joint is usually uncomfortable or painful. There is often stiffness in the joint on arising in the morning or after sitting for more than a few minutes at one time. The areas of pain may also feel warm to touch. Arthritis may involve one or many joints at one time so that other areas of the body may also be painful. There may be difficulty using the joint for daily activities because of pain or stiffness. This may make it difficult to walk, climb stairs, or dress and undress.

If you notice pain or stiffness which lasts more than a few days or is severe then you should contact your physician. Other problems may mimic the pain of arthritis and may require specific treatment.

Discussion and examination are important for diagnosis. Then x-rays of the areas involved and blood tests may be ordered. If there is swelling in the joint, a simple procedure in the office under local anesthetic can remove fluid for analysis. This helps in diagnosis since different kinds of arthritis cause different changes in the joint fluid.

Treatment usually includes moist heat, rest, and at some point gradual addition of exercises to keep the joint flexible and the muscles strong. Medications commonly used are those called anti-inflammatory drugs. These attempt to decrease the inflammation of arthritis and related problems which then decreases the pain, swelling and stiffness. They usually take at least a few days to work. These may give excellent relief but there are some possible side effects. Be sure you talk with your physician before you take these. This group of medications is discussed on page 158. If the problem remains severe your physician may refer you to a specialist in arthritis such as a rheumatologist or an orthopedic surgeon.

Leg Pain Due to Thrombophlebitis

An important cause of leg pain is thrombophlebitis (blood clot in the veins of the leg or pelvis). It is important to be recognized and treated as early as possible. The chance of thrombophlebitis seems to increase with age. It is most common in persons who have another medical problem, especially after surgery. It is also common in persons who have heart disease, cancer, or are inactive. Some researchers have found that thrombophlebitis may be more common in women who take oral contraceptives. These and other causes seem in some way to increase the chance of clots forming in the veins of the legs and pelvis. The most dangerous form of thrombophlebitis happens in veins that are deep in the legs and pelvis. In these cases, blood clots may move to the lungs (pulmonary embolus) and cause serious illness and death. Treatment is very effective to prevent pulmonary embolus if started early.

You may feel nothing. You may feel pain and tightness in the calf or thigh. Thrombophlebitis usually happens on one side although it is possible to involve both legs at the same time. The pain is usually constant but may be made worse by standing or walking.

There may be no visible changes. There may be swelling in the lower leg and foot or tenderness on pressure in the calf. You may notice redness over the lower leg. These changes may happen only in the calf and lower leg or may extend to the thigh. Since you may see no changes even if there is thrombophlebitis present, don't wait for visible signs to see your physician.

After discussion and examination, your physician may schedule a test of the veins in the legs to decide whether thrombophlebitis is present. The tests measure the flow of blood or visualize the veins to help decide if thrombophlebitis is present.

Elevation of the leg with bedrest, other measures for pain, and medications to prevent further blood clot formation are needed in thrombophlebitis in the deep veins of the legs, thighs, and pelvis. This often requires hospitalization for 5-10 days in order to give medication by vein. Oral forms of these medications such as warfarin (Coumadin) may be required for several months after the initial treatment. Treatment of any of the above underlying medical problems is also important.

Disease of the Arteries

Another cause of pain in the legs is due to atherosclerosis in the arteries which supply blood to the thighs, legs, and feet. This develops over many years and is more common in those persons who smoke cigarettes, have hypertension or high blood cholesterol. See the discussion of other risk factors for atherosclerosis on page 27. As the atherosclerosis worsens over years the arteries become narrowed and blood supply is limited to the legs and feet.

Discomfort in the legs, especially the calf, is common. The discomfort usually is first noticed as a tightness, cramp, or aching pain or weakness in the calf muscles which happens when walking. It stops after a few minutes of rest. After the discomfort leaves, walking can be resumed again. Often there is a fairly predictable distance in walking before the discomfort happens. The term for this discomfort is intermittent claudication. When these feelings happen your physician should be contacted.

As the blood supply decreases even more, the discomfort may become more painful and may happen even when not active. The pain can become very severe and may prevent sleep and activity. Ulcers or breaks in the skin may appear and may be painful. If there is no treatment then the loss of blood supply may worsen and gangrene may develop in the toes and foot. Immediate medical care is needed.

Early in the course there may be no changes which are easily seen. When the early feelings happen you should seek medical care. Later on the foot may be pale or reddened, hair over the toes may disappear, and ulcers or broken skin may happen. These are late changes. Don't wait for these visible changes to see a physician. Your family physician or a vascular surgeon can help guide you to proper treatment which may save the foot from amputation.

After discussion and examination your physician will have a reasonable idea of the problem. Tests may include evaluation of the arteries in the legs by ultrasonic methods using a Doppler system. This is painless and is often helpful in diagnosis. Arteriogram with x-ray after dye injection is still the most accurate way of finding the areas of blockage in these arteries. Since these problems can be caused by diseases other than atherosclerosis, your physician may plan other tests to be sure no other problems are present.

Stopping cigarette smoking, protection of the feet and legs from injury, early treatment of infection, and removal of risk factors for atherosclerosis are important. Medications do not cure the problem but there are some now available which may be helpful. In some cases surgery of the arteries is needed to improve the blood supply. If all treatments are not helpful then surgery and amputation of the involved toes, foot or lower leg may be necessary. Treatment must be individualized and will be guided by your physician.

Leg Pain—Other Causes

Another common cause of leg pain is pain caused by abnormalities in the nerves of the legs. This can be caused by irritation of the nerves in the lower part of the back (lumbar spine) as they travel to supply the legs. This can also be caused by irritation of the smaller nerve endings throughout the feet and lower legs. Both problems can cause pain, numbness, tingling and other abnormal sensations in the legs. These are not the only cause of nerve-related pain in the legs although they are the most common.

The sciatic nerve extends from the lower portion of the spinal cord to supply the entire lower extremity. Pressure or irritation of this nerve causes pain called *sciatica*. This may cause pain in the lower back which extends down to the leg, most commonly felt in the back of the thigh and down to the calf and foot. Other feelings such as numbness, tingling, a feeling like "hot water pouring down the leg" are common.

If you have these or similar feelings you should contact your physician. If the pain is severe or awakens you at night, if it is worse when you cough or sneeze, or if you notice any change in your bowel or bladder habits you should contact your physician immediately.

There are many different causes of sciatica. This can be confusing because not all cases of pain in the lower back and leg are actually caused by true sciatica. There are many other problems which mimic this pain which are not actually caused by pressure or irritation on the sciatic nerve. Many of these other causes are less serious even though they may cause real discomfort.

After discussion and examination, x-rays of the lower back or other areas involved may be planned. Depending on what evidence is present and the severity of the pain, other tests available include computed tomographic scan of the lumbar spine, magnetic resonance imaging of the lumbar spine, specific testing of individual nerves and myelography. Each of these tests may help your physician decide where the problem is and the exact cause of the nerve abnormality. The causes are numerous including arthritis, disease of the disc which separates the bones of the spine (ruptured or herniated disc), infection, injury, and other problems.

Treatment depends on finding the specific underlying cause if possible. Some relief may happen after bedrest and with medications for pain. Try to follow your physician's advice. This can be a frustrating problem because there is often no excellent quick remedy available. Weeks may be required for improvement after the more serious causes of this problem are eliminated by testing. If improvement does not follow then your physician may refer you to a specialist such as a neurosurgeon, orthopedic surgeon, or neurologist.

Leg pain can also be caused by irritation of the smaller nerves or nerve endings which supply the feet, legs, and thighs. Rather than pressure or irritation on the larger nerve near the spinal cord, there may be irritation of the nerve or more than one nerve farther along its course toward the foot. These problems in the peripheral nerves are called *peripheral neuropathy*.

Most common is irritation of the smaller nerve endings in the feet and lower legs. The discomfort may be pain, burning, coldness, tightness, numbness or may be more difficult to describe. It may come on gradually or suddenly and may or may not be constant. It may not be made worse by activity but may interfere with sleep. Any portion of the foot, leg or thigh may be affected, but most common are problems in both feet and lower legs. If you notice any persistent unexplained discomfort as described in the feet or legs or if you notice weakness in the muscles of the lower extremities you should contact your physician.

When the discomfort begins there are usually no visible changes in the feet or legs. Much later there may be changes in the skin color or texture. Weakness may be present in muscles. Medical care should not wait for visible signs.

Discussion and examination will be followed by tests including blood tests to look for internal problems such as diabetes mellitus, arthritis and related diseases, and many other possible causes. Specific tests of nerve function called nerve conduction studies and related tests may be ordered. The cause is not found in many cases. Your physician can guide you and may refer you to a specialist such as a neurologist. Treatment depends on the cause of the peripheral neuropathy. If no cause is found, some medications are available which often give relief.

Leg Ulcers

Pain in the feet and legs may be caused by ulcers in which there is loss of an area of skin. The ulcer may appear as a shallow or deep hole in the skin and may be small, only a few millimeters, or may be much larger. Ulcerations may be painful, especially when narrowing of the arteries is also present from diseases such as atherosclerosis. Atherosclerosis and narrowing of the arteries often causes ulcers around the toes, between the toes, and around the heels.

Ulcers on the ankles and lower legs also happen in disease of the veins which return the blood from the feet back toward the heart. These ulcers may have less pain than ulcers which happen when there is blockage of the arteries. Other internal problems may also be associated with leg ulcers.

All ulcers of the legs and feet are important and should have medical treatment, whether there is pain or not. It is important that the ulcer be treated early and that the underlying cause is found and treated.

These are a few of the most common causes of leg pain. All of the causes of leg pain are not listed here. Don't try to diagnose your own cause of leg pain. If the pain is severe or persistent, contact your physician to allow the earliest possible proper diagnosis and treatment.

■ LUMPS IN THE NECK

Lumps in the neck are a common cause of alarm to patients of all ages. It is most likely a lymph node enlargement due to an infection arising in the nose or throat area. It represents the body's attempt to prevent the infection from spreading through the body. The lumps or nodes disappear after the infection; however, some do not disappear completely and may remain enlarged for years. On occasion, it may be more serious, and for this reason any lump or lymph node in the neck that remains for greater than two weeks should be seen by your physician to rule out a tumor. A lump that increases and decreases in size, particularly with regard to eating, may be salivary gland origin. This swelling may be with or without pain. It should be checked by your physician.

■ MACULAR DEGENERATION

As people grow older, a decrease in sight may be due to deterioration of the central area of the retina called the macula. Many feel that long-term exposure to sunlight contributes to this condition. Heredity and nutrition are also thought to play a role.

The first symptom of this condition is a decrease in visual acuity that cannot be corrected with glasses. A thorough retinal examination is warranted. Patients with macular degeneration can also experience sudden changes in their vision which cause them to see straight lines as "waves." If this occurs, evaluation by an ophthalmologist as soon as possible is recommended, as total loss of central vision is possible. A laser treatment may be necessary to avoid this serious complication.

People with macular degeneration do not usually lose their side vision and are able to see well enough to take care of themselves, performing work that does not require keen vision. The ophthalmologist has a number of low vision aids which may enhance the vision that remains and therefore help the patient lead a more productive life.

■ MOUTH

The most common problems in the mouth are benign in origin and usually spontaneously clear. Irritation of the gums, tongue, or cheek, by poor fitting dentures is a common complaint, and your dentist should be consulted. The enlargement of the taste buds at the base of the tongue is not a danger but is usually due to irritation by tobacco or a virus. The angles of the mouth may develop reddened areas that are sometimes painful. This is usually due to decreased vitamin B, yeast infection, or constant moisture in the corner of the lips from licking the corner as a habit.

The mouth heals very rapidly due to its excellent blood supply. After any injury such as a burn from hot food or injury from a utensil in eating there should be marked improvement in 10–14 days. If improvement does not happen during this time, you should see your dentist. Other warning signs to be aware of include severe pain, tenderness to touch, swelling, or fever. If any of these are present in mouth injuries or mouth soreness, contact your dentist.

Mouth Ulcers (Aphthous Ulcers)

Aphthous ulcers or mouth ulcers are very common. They are spots with white centers and red margins almost like a crater edge. Customarily, they appear rapidly and are painful for 4 to 10 days. They can be treated with various over-the-counter preparations. On occasion, a physician may be needed to prescribe an antibiotic. Environmental stress appears as a significant contribution to this disorder.

If ulcers are generalized throughout the mouth there may be other medical problems present. These include other underlying diseases, diet, and reactions to medications.

■ OBESITY (OVERWEIGHT)

Although there are many jokes about persons who are overweight, there is now good evidence that it carries a higher risk for medical problems and death. If obesity is defined as 20 percent over desirable body weight, it can be shown that this weight or higher raises the risks of certain specific diseases. In most cases a reduction of weight to desirable levels also lowers the risk of these diseases.

Some researchers have found hypertension to be almost 3 times higher in obese compared to nonobese persons. The risk was higher up to age 44, and remained twice as high after age 45 in obese persons. Diabetes mellitus was almost 3 times higher in overweight persons in one study. Coronary heart disease has been found to be more frequent in obese persons in some studies although the relationship is not as strong as in hypertension. But it should be remembered that hypertension and diabetes mellitus are definite risk factors for coronary heart disease.

Higher mortality rates in obese persons from several different kinds of cancer have been found by researchers. These include cancer of the colon, prostate, and rectum in obese men. Women who were obese had more frequent cancer of the gallbladder, breast, uterus, and ovaries.

It was found by researchers that the greater the degree of overweight, the higher the excess death rate seems to be from all causes.

Look at Table 27 on page 95 for desirable or ideal body weight. See where your own situation fits for body height, weight, and build. If your body weight is 20 percent or higher above desirable weight then you should consider a weight loss program. If your body weight is 100 pounds or more above desirable then your situation is extremely serious and weight loss is mandatory.

Experts also tell us that weight loss down to desirable levels should be considered even if less than 20 percent overweight if certain diseases are also present. These include diabetes mellitus, hypertension, high blood cholesterol and high blood triglycerides. Many specialists would also suggest weight loss to desirable levels in coronary heart disease, emphysema and chronic bronchitis, and arthritis in the hips, knees and spine.

If you are overweight, and especially if you are more than 20 percent over your desirable body weight, talk with your physician. Make plans to begin a reasonable weight loss program safely. If other medical problems are present they may affect the rate and success of your weight loss. A reasonable diet combined with a regular exercise program is usually successful and fairly painless. Before a diet and exercise program is begun, however, it is necessary to be sure that it is safe.

■ OSTEOARTHRITIS (also see Arthritis)

Osteoarthritis is the most common kind of arthritis. It is more common in older persons, especially after age 50. It may happen earlier, especially if there has been an injury to a joint. An example is the athlete who injures the knee and later develops osteoarthritis in that knee. It is most common in joints that bear more weight over the years such as the knees, hips, and lower part of the spine. It usually comes on gradually over months or years. Some persons notice a few minutes of stiffness in the involved joint when they arise in the morning. Except for the pain and stiffness in the involved joints the person usually feels quite well. There is no unusual tiredness or fatigue.

The joint or joints involved are usually painful and swollen. There may be warmth in the joint to touch. There may be difficulty in activities such as walking when the knee or hip are affected. There is often little or no pain when not trying to walk.

X-rays show typical changes to help diagnose osteoarthritis. A few other tests may be helpful including blood tests to help eliminate other causes of arthritis and examination of a sample of joint fluid.

The goals of treatment are to control pain and to allow the arthritis patient to be able to move around and do as many desired activities as possible.

Treatment includes the use of moist heat and exercises to keep the joints flexible and to strengthen the muscles which support the joints. Anti-inflammatory medications often give improvement in the pain and stiffness and may allow much better activity and mobility. Most persons are able to find a medication which gives good relief with no significant side effects. Local injection of a joint or surgery may also be needed at times.

In severe cases, total joint replacement of the joint by an orthopedic surgeon may give excellent relief of pain and allow improvement in activity. This has been most successful in the hip so far with results of replacement of the knee improving over recent years.

■ OSTEOPOROSIS (See page 55.)

■ PALPITATIONS

Palpitations is the term many persons refer to when they feel rapid, irregular or more forceful heart beat than usual. Some persons feel as if their heart "skipped a beat." Palpitations can happen in normal persons with no other underlying heart disease and no other medical problems. Palpitations may also be a sign of more serious disease, including heart disease as well as other medical problems. If you feel frequent or severe rapid, irregular or slow heart rate or heart skipping then it is safest to contact your physician. Tests will be done to be sure that no heart disease and no other underlying medical problems are present. In most persons who are otherwise healthy no other problems are found. However, to be safe it is best to discuss the problem with your physician.

■ PNEUMONIA

Pneumonia refers to inflammation in the lung. There are many different causes of pneumonia. The most common causes are infections. Infections may be caused by bacteria, viruses and other diseases.

Pneumonia may follow an upper respiratory infection or "flu-like" illness. There may be cough, fever, sputum or phlegm on coughing, shortness of breath and at times sharp pains in the chest when a deep breath is taken. However, some or all of these common signs may not be present. This is especially common in older persons or in persons who have other underlying medical problems. For example, in elderly patients the only feeling may be pain in the stomach or abdomen. Fever may not be very prominent in older patients.

If there is a persistent "cold," cough, fever, or if shortness of breath or chest pains happen—especially if any of these follow another infection, you should contact your physician. Tests including a chest x-ray can help make the diagnosis. Then proper treatment of the pneumonia (or other problem) can begin.

Immunization for one of the most common types of pneumonia is available. Pneumococcal pneumonia can be more serious with complications including death, especially in persons over age 65 and in those with other problems such as heart disease. The immunization now available is effective and lowers the risk of this infection. One injection is recommended and does not need to be repeated. It is recommended for persons over age 65 and those with other chronic illnesses such as heart disease, lung disease, diabetes mellitus, and those who for other reasons have an increased risk of pneumococcal infection. To be safe, check with your physician to see if this is needed and safe in your own situation.

Influenza immunization is also recommended for those over 65 and those with chronic diseases as above. Yearly influenza immunizations lower the risk for serious influenza infection including pneumonia. Other recommendations for immunization for influenza are discussed on page 63.

■ POLYMYALGIA RHEUMATICA

Polymyalgia rheumatica is a strange-sounding disease which affects persons mainly over 60 but almost always over age 50. The cause is unknown. It often happens in a person who was previously quite well. There is a sudden or gradual onset of severe pain and stiffness in the muscles around the shoulders and upper arms and the hips and thighs. Usually there is no swelling in the joints. There is severe fatigue and severe stiffness on arising in the morning. The pain is often so severe that it is hard to turn over in bed at night! There may be mild fever, weight loss and poor appetite.

There is little to see except a very uncomfortable person. There is usually prominent tenderness to touch over the upper arms, shoulders, and over the thighs and hips.

In addition to discussion and examination, blood tests to look for other diseases are usually done. The most useful test is the sedimentation rate which is an old blood test and is usually very abnormally elevated in polymyalgia rheumatica. It is important to look for other medical problems as well which may mimic this disease. Especially important is temporal arteritis which is discussed on page 227.

Treatment usually requires low doses of prednisone or other cortisone derivative. There is usually very quick improvement and return to feeling nearly normal over a few days. Then the medication is slowly decreased over a period of months as long as improvement continues. There are usually no permanent effects of the polymyalgia rheumatica such as crippling or deformity after it leaves.

■ PROSTATE DISEASES

The prostate gland is present in men at the base of the bladder around the urethra (the tube that conducts urine out of the bladder). The prostate produces fluid that is mixed with sperm. The size of the prostate commonly increases with age. Problems of the prostate are common in men over age 50. By age 65 to 70, it is common for men to develop symptoms such as decreased force in the urine stream, frequency of urination, difficulty starting and stopping urination and arising several times each night to empty the bladder. Eventually enlargement of the prostate may cause complete blockage of urine flow.

Not all men with enlargement of the prostate develop infection or obstruction of urine flow. Feelings and signs of urinary tract infection or obstruction need further evaluation. A change in the pattern of urination, blood in the urine, or urinary leakage requires urologic evaluation. This often includes discussion, physical examination, test of urine specimen, intravenous pyelogram (IVP), and cystoscopy. In cystoscopy, the bladder is examined using a fiberoptic instrument. When blockage of urine flow occurs, a surgical procedure called TURP (trans urethral resection of the prostate) is necessary to allow satisfactory voiding. This is one of the most common operations performed by urologists.

In some cases a biopsy of the prostate gland may be needed to be sure that no cancer is present. The prostate gland may be enlarged but have no cancer. This is called benign prostatic hypertrophy and usually requires no further specific treatment.

The type of treatment when prostate cancer is present depends on the severity of the cancer and whether it is confined to the prostate itself. Other important factors are the age of the patient, the general health, and the patient's choice in treatment. In many patients over 75-years-old, prostate cancer is discovered but shows no progression. Prostate cancer often takes many years to develop and may be very slow growing, especially in the elderly. Treatment must be individualized depending on all these factors. Treatment available includes surgery, radiation therapy, and medication.

A 76-year-old man was seen recently because his physician noticed a small knot on his prostate during a routine examination. He had no other unusual signs or feelings. Test of urine and blood and x-rays of the kidney and bladder were normal. Since about half of these nodules in the prostate may be cancer, a simple biopsy of the nodule was performed. The result showed cancer of the prostate. Because of his age and a heart problem, surgery was not performed. He was treated with radiation therapy as an outpatient. Five years later he continues to be free of disease.

The results in this patient were excellent because of early detection of the cancer which allowed effective treatment. He will continue to be checked about every six months to be sure no cancer returns.

■ RHEUMATOID ARTHRITIS (also see Arthritis)

Rheumatoid arthritis is a problem in which the linings of the joints become inflamed. The cause is not known. It is more common in women than men and can happen at almost any age. It usually comes on gradually with pain, stiffness and swelling in the hands, wrists, elbows, shoulders, knees, ankles, or feet. There is usually bothersome stiffness in all the joints on arising in the morning. Fatigue is usually prominent. In fact, most patients complain about fatigue as much or more than the actual joint pain! Fever, weight loss, and other problems may happen. Rheumatoid arthritis can cause so many different problems that it may be confused with many other diseases.

The joints may be painful, swollen and warm to touch. Muscles may become smaller and weaker. The pain and stiffness cause difficulty performing daily activities at work and at home. It may become difficult to dress or to use food utensils. In severe cases walking as well as most other activities required for daily living may be severely limited.

Discussion and examination will usually be followed by a few blood tests and x-rays. In most cases there is a fairly typical combination of findings which allows the diagnosis to be made. The blood test which is widely used to help in diagnosis is the rheumatoid factor. This is present in 70 to 80 percent of patients with rheumatoid arthritis. (Rheumatoid factor may also be present in problems *other* than rheumatoid arthritis.)

Treatment of rheumatoid arthritis is aimed at control of pain and maintaining use of the joints. In the majority of persons the joint pain and stiffness can be controlled. The goal should be to have enough control so that the person affected is able to be comfortable and to do the desired daily activities. Five percent or less of rheumatoid arthritis patients have a severe crippling course. With treatment most affected persons are able to view rheumatoid arthritis as being inconvenient but not terrible or devastating. Most persons can continue to do most of the activities they choose with some modifications at times. It is thought that many times the best control may happen if control of the rheumatoid arthritis is gained within the first year or so of the beginning. Therefore to have a better chance at control of the arthritis try to have the earliest and most effective treatment possible.

Treatment includes moist heat and exercises to keep the joints flexible and strengthen the muscles that support the joints. Proper rest will help the fatigue. Anti-inflammatory medications often improve the joint pain, swelling, stiffness, and may improve the fatigue and stiffness of the joints in the morning. Anti-inflammatory drugs include aspirin and other medications. See the discussion of anti-inflammatory medications on page 158.

The majority of rheumatoid arthritis patients can control their disease adequately with a basic program such as this. If none of the available anti-inflammatory medications prove effective then there is a second group of medications available which may help suppress the arthritis. This group of medicines includes gold compounds, methotrexate, penicillamine and others. These may be extremely effective but take longer to work. They may have side effects and are given under close medical supervision.

The treatment of serious arthritis such as rheumatoid arthritis must be individualized. Your physician can guide you to proper care and may ask that you be seen by a rheumatologist, an arthritis specialist.

■ RHINITIS—CAUSED BY MEDICATION

Medication rhinitis is due to chemical irritation for prolonged use of over-the-counter nasal spray. The nasal spray junkie requires with time increasing amounts of spray to obtain an open nasal passage. In the nose this produces an irritation of the lining with swelling, further blockage and, in some cases, even nasal discharge. A substitute of over-the-counter saline nasal spray will benefit. If, however, it is not helpful, a visit to your physician or specialist will provide relief.

■ SEXUAL PROBLEMS (SEXUAL DYSFUNCTION)

Sexual dysfunction refers to the feeling of unsatisfactory sexual activity. When this happens in men your physician or urologist will plan an evaluation. When this happens in females your physician or gynecologist will plan further studies.

One of the most common problems causing sexual dysfunction in men is impotence, which refers to unsatisfactory or incomplete erection. Many men feel uncomfortable discussing impotence which may cause delay in adequate medical treatment. Early diagnosis and treatment is much more effective and is usually easier and less expensive.

Impotence is often thought to be a condition of old men with difficulty achieving and maintaining an erection due to old age or psychological problems. In the last twenty years medical evidence has been found that in many of these cases there is actually an underlying medical problem instead of psychological problem or old age. Two of the most common examples are impotence found in some diabetic patients and impotence caused by medications used in hypertension. As men get older the ability to achieve and maintain an erection does not necessarily disappear. There is some evidence that it may be slower or less frequent. Men well into their eighties may be quite capable of having satisfactory erection and sexual activity. Therefore when impotence or other unsatisfactory activity happens then evaluation is important to be sure that no other medical problems are present. Several factors are important in achieving erection. If there is excess stress, fear or anxiety then erection may be more difficult. This may be caused in part by changes in the action of some hormones. It has been estimated that 15 to 20 percent of persons with impotence are caused by such problems. At times failure at sexual activity may cause so much anxiety that it may aggravate later attempts and sexual activity. The problem of impotence should definitely not be assumed to be psychological until thorough evaluation is complete.

After discussion and physical examination certain tests may be planned such as a blood test to measure the level of male hormone (testosterone) and other tests to be sure no other medical problems are present. An accurate record of medications is important since many can contribute to impotence. Hardening and narrowing of the arteries (atherosclerosis) can cause decrease in blood flow to pelvic organs and may cause difficulty in erection.

Medical problems which affect nerve function to the pelvic organs may also cause impotence. The most common example is in persons with diabetes mellitus. The exact causes of the changes of the nerve function in these persons is not very well understood. These nerve abnormalities may affect other organs throughout the body as well. Also, atherosclerosis is more common in diabetics which may contribute to impotence.

In most cases impotence due only to low male hormone levels is less common. In these cases the problem may be caused by a disease in the pituitary gland, thyroid gland or testicle. Failure of the testicle to produce normal male hormone level can be caused by medication, blood vessel disease, surgery, injury or other problem affecting the testicle. Age alone does not necessarily cause a decrease in male hormone level.

Disease in the prostate gland can cause impotence. Inflammation, infection, or surgery in the prostate can all be a cause of impotence.

Any major injury or surgery in the pelvis area can cause damage to the nerves that supply the penis and may result in impotence. For example, a seventeen-year-old man suffered a serious fracture of the pelvis in an auto accident. Permanent nerve damage caused difficulty in achieving satisfactory erections. In such cases other treatment and techniques are available to improve sexual function. A surgical procedure in this case allowed the patient to have satisfactory sexual activity. This man has since been the father of three children.

Prostate surgery in some cases can cause impotence. The type of major prostate surgery which leads to impotence is complete removal of the prostate gland. This surgery is used less commonly today except in certain cases of prostate cancer. This depends on the individual situation. Newer techniques have been reported which may decrease the chance of impotence after this surgery in the future.

Treatment for impotence caused by such surgery or by other problems is available. These treatments include medications, injections and prosthetic surgery of the penis in which a prosthesis is inserted into the penis and usually allows satisfactory sexual function. Most patients are quite satisfied after such surgery for treatment of impotence. Since each person is different, specific problems and questions can be answered by your urologist.

■ SHORTNESS OF BREATH

Shortness of breath (the medical term is dyspnea) causes a feeling of breathlessness or a sense of "not enough air" out of proportion to activity. For example, shortness of breath which happens when you are not active or with little physical activity is not normal. If you notice shortness of breath with much less activity than you have experienced before, or especially if you become short of breath while not active, then you should see your physician. If you awaken at night short of breath you should contact your physician. Don't wait for other signs or changes.

Tests will be ordered after your discussion and physical examination by your physician. Tests may include chest x-ray, tests of lung function and oxygen levels in the blood if lung disease is suspected. Other tests may be ordered to evaluate possible heart disease including electrocardiogram and other tests. Treatment depends on the cause of the shortness of breath.

■ SKIN CHANGES

Skin changes seem to increase with the increase in sun or wind exposure and with the aging process. Some of these changes are entirely benign and can be treated with topical medications. Aging spots are particularly benefited by the use of topical application of bleaching creams or, in some cases, by physician application of liquid nitrogen. Some changes require only to be seen and are so characteristic in appearance that no biopsy is necessary. These can be treated by appropriate medications, or may require surface freezing or shaving in the physician's office. On occasion, electrosurgery or chemical cauterization is necessary with a minimum of discomfort. On occasion the skin changes require a biopsy and more involved treatment may be required. If it is a skin cancer, the key in treatment is the removal of the cancer under microscopic check. In some cases, particularly in the face and neck region, local reconstruction using grafts or local flaps are necessary and these can be done in a well-trained surgeon's office, under a local anesthetic with minimal discomfort and inconvenience.

One of the most important ways to care for the skin is prevention of sun damage. Sun damage actually begins the first time that we are exposed to ultraviolet light. Damage accumulates in the lower layers of the skin. When skin is unable to store any further damage, the changes become visible on the surface. Looking in a mirror you are able to see changes that have happened to your skin from the sun.

You may see thickness of the skin in certain areas such as the face and arms. There may be enlarged blood vessels in those areas, especially in the face. There may also be areas with more or less pigment which appear darker or lighter. There may be small growths which are usually harmless. (See warning signs on page 220.)

If you look closely, the skin usually covered by clothes or bathing suit is softer and younger-looking. Prolonged exposure to the sun causes more breakdown of the collagen layers of the skin and makes these changes happen more rapidly.

The damage from the sun accumulates. It is now a routine recommendation that even young children wear a sunscreen with a sun protective factor (SPF) of 15 or higher. This will protect the average person almost totally from the harmful rays of the sun and can help preserve youthfulness in the skin. Protective clothing is also acceptable and may be used along with sunscreens for more complete protection.

Dryness of the skin is common and is often worse with frequent hot shower or bath during the winter. Cooler water for bath and shower in the winter and more frequent use of body lotions and oils may help prevent dryness of the skin. In warm and humid environments such as the summer regular bathing helps reduce sweating and body odor. Proper care of the skin can help you maintain healthy skin.

Fair-skinned persons with prolonged sun exposure are more likely to have enlarged blood vessels over the face, especially in the center or flush area of the face. If the appearance of these are bothersome to the person then treatment is available which may help eradicate these veins.

"Spider" veins are enlarged veins which occur commonly over the legs. They are often purple, snake-like and may be seen in young as well as older persons. These can be treated in several ways. An electric current can be used in a procedure which coagulates the vein. Also, a substance may be injected into the vein which causes inflammation and obliteration of the vein. This is called sclerosis and is one of the most widely used treatments. A newer treatment is the use of lasers. A new tunable dye laser is now available that can produce resolution of the unwanted veins without damage to the overlying skin. The procedure is nearly painless but is expensive.

Common problems seen by dermatologists are pigment (darkened) spots on the face and back of the hands. These may become prominent although they are usually benign (not malignant or cancer). Treatment includes bleaching creams although the results are slow to appear. These areas may be frozen with liquid nitrogen, but this may leave the area lighter in appearance.

Retin-A is currently being used for wrinkling and for pigment spots over the face. Retin-A must be used under the supervision of your physician or dermatologist. In some persons the results are remarkable with a much younger appearance after one year's treatment. Retin-A may make some persons more sun-sensitive. In these persons sunscreens are recommended for use along with Retin-A.

■ SKIN CANCER

There are basically three types of skin cancer for most of us to be concerned about. A *basal cell carcinoma* is often a pearly type of growth found in sun-exposed areas. These may bleed easily with contact. They may grow very slowly over years and produce no feelings or other changes to suggest that they are a troublesome growth. Basal cell carcinomas do not usually spread to other areas of the body, but they may cause damage locally including loss of the structure of a portion of the ear or nose if not treated.

The second most common skin cancer is *squamous cell carcinoma*. If these arise in an area of previously sun-damaged skin they are less likely to spread than those that arise from normal skin. This type of growth may happen more suddenly than a basal cell carcinoma and may be more hazardous. These need to be removed as early as possible.

The third and most feared of the skin cancers is *malignant melanoma*. Melanomas may arise from an existing mole or may be new. The success of early treatment depends on the depth of the penetration of the melanoma into the skin and its spread. Removed early, then melanoma has an excellent chance for a cure. If not treated early, treatment may not be as effective. *Any time a new growth appears on the skin it is reasonable to see your physician for an evaluation.*

■ SKIN MOLES (NEVI)

Skin moles or nevi are dark or light growths which may appear any place on the skin. It has recently been found that moles in sun-exposed areas have a higher chance of malignant change. There are three warning signs for skin moles:

1. A sudden change in size of the mole
2. A sudden change of color
3. A persistent irritation such as itching, bleeding, or crumbling.

There is often a change in a mole which (if noticed early) will allow the mole to be removed early before it becomes a cancer and before it extends to other areas of the body. Try to observe the moles on your skin and notice any changes. Some persons with a large number of moles may find it helpful to see a dermatologist yearly or other regular visit for help in decisions about changes in moles.

Remember, these suggestions are not designed for self-diagnosis. These are to aid in deciding whether a change in the skin warrants a visit to the physician or dermatologist. If you are not sure about a change in the skin then you should see your physician for advice.

■ SKIN INFECTIONS

Skin infections are common, especially in warmer climates. One of the most frequently seen skin infections is ringworm, a type of fungus. Athlete's foot and jock itch are common examples, especially in men. It is believed that sweating contributes to these fungus infections in the feet and the groin area. In these infections there are itching, redness, and a border which may gradually enlarge and may appear like a ring. Ringworm infections are usually not highly contagious. They can be treated with cream, ointment, powders or other medications.

A yeast-like fungus can infect the body folds such as under the breasts, between the buttocks and under folds of fat. This may also involve the lips and nails. This type of yeast is produced by Candida and is the same cause of thrush in a baby's mouth, diaper rash in babies, and some fingernail infections in persons who frequently have their hands in water.

Herpes simplex is the fever blister virus. This is a contagious infection. When found in the groin it is often called genital herpes. There are newer medications for the treatment of both the fever blister type of herpes and the genital type of herpes.

Shingles or herpes zoster is a problem caused by a virus. This is the same virus which causes chicken pox in younger persons. It commonly becomes active again in older persons. This results in a bang-like or "shingle" of blisters along the path of a nerve. Early diagnosis by a physician may allow the use of new medications to help relieve the pain which may be long-lasting.

Bacteria can cause infection in the skin. These most commonly include Staphylococcus and Streptococcus infections. Superficial infection may occur such as impetigo. Deeper abscesses may also happen in any area of the body. Usually antibiotics help to eradicate the bacteria responsible for the infection.

Other skin problems can be caused by certain types of insect bites, various types of body lice, and the mite of scabies. Close living contacts such as in nursing homes and institutions may make these more likely. Clothing and furniture may even help spread these problems. If there is sudden onset of itching with no apparent rash then a problem of this type may be present and advice from your physician would be recommended.

◼ SNORING

Snoring is a result of vibration of the soft tissues of the throat and palate caused by deep inspiration of air. It is more common in individuals who sleep with their mouths open (usually due to partial nasal obstruction), exhausted individuals, or those under the influence of sedative medications or alcohol. Snoring can result in reducing the oxygen level in the bloodstream in some individuals with disturbance of sleep resulting in constant daily symptoms of tiredness. (See the discussion of daytime sleepiness on page 199.) A visit to the physician would be appropriate to evaluate the cause of the snoring which is often treatable.

◼ SORE THROAT (PHARYNGITIS)

Sore throat is usually due to infection by a virus or bacteria. A swab culture of the throat may be necessary to determine its cause. A rapid test to determine if streptococcal throat infection is present is sometimes done. If tonsils are present, then their infection (tonsillitis) can cause the sore throat. In general, if the pain is mild and temperature is under 100, then acetaminophen, increased fluids, and rest will suffice. If not improved quickly or if there is difficulty breathing, then a call to your physician is in order. In individuals under 25, mononucleosis must be considered, especially if there is an enlarged node in the neck. Remember that any sore throat, no matter what the age of the patient, must be seen if it lasts over 14 days.

◼ STROKE (CEREBROVASCULAR ACCIDENT)

A sudden attack which often causes weakness or paralysis of the face, hand, arm, foot, or leg is a stroke. Many other feelings and problems can happen in a stroke, including difficulty or loss of speech, loss of feeling in an arm or leg, loss of consciousness, loss of vision, unsteadiness, and others.

Strokes can quickly disable a person who previously had normal activity. The most common type of stroke is blockage of an artery in the brain. The problems this causes depend on which artery is blocked. If the artery supplied the portion of the brain that controls speech, then speech will be affected. If the artery supplied a portion of the brain which controls movements of the muscles of the leg, then the leg may be weak or paralyzed. Any of the functions of the brain may be affected depending on the artery involved. Certain patterns are common, such as the combination of weakness or paralysis of the left hand, left arm, and left leg and foot. Or, weakness of the right hand and arm, right foot and leg, and loss of speech. Weakness of the muscles of the face may also happen. The most common underlying cause of stroke is atherosclerosis and narrowing of the blood vessels in the brain or in the neck leading to the brain. Atherosclerosis develops over many years and is most common in those persons who have the risk factors of hypertension, high blood cholesterol, and cigarette smoking. (See the discussion of risk factors and how to control them in Chapter 2.) Control or removal of risk factors can greatly lower your own chance of stroke.

Strokes may be preceded by temporary episodes in which there is numbness or weakness of a hand, arm, foot, leg, or one side of the face. These episodes usually last a few minutes but may last longer (up to 24 hours) and go away completely. An episode is called a transient ischemic attack (TIA). Researchers have found that the most dangerous time is immediately after the first episode. Some researchers have found that 7 percent of these persons may have a stroke within 24 hours. All persons with these transient ischemic attacks (TIAs) do not develop a stroke, but the risk of future stroke remains higher after the episode.

Other causes of strokes include bleeding in the brain which may be caused by hypertension and abnormalities of the arteries. Certain types of heart disease as well as other less common medical problems may lead to a stroke.

After a discussion and examination a computed tomographic (CT) scan of the head is used in most cases and will help your physician decide the cause and any further treatment needed. Tests to look for atherosclerosis of arteries in the neck may be planned. Other tests are available depending on the individual situation. Plans will be made to look for underlying causes such as atherosclerosis and its risk factors. This will include blood tests and other studies.

Treatment will depend on the situation. When stroke is suspected then hospitalization for proper diagnosis and treatment is often necessary. Diagnosis includes assessing the extent of the stroke and finding the underlying cause. Treatment includes treatment of the acute stroke to prevent complications as well as treatment of the underlying problem for prevention of future strokes.

Possible treatments for transient ischemic attacks include removal or control of risk factors for atherosclerosis, certain medications, and at times surgery. Risk factor control and removal is discussed in Chapter 2. Medications used include aspirin and dipyridamole which are given alone or in combination. These medications affect platelets which are cells in the blood which affect blood clotting. There is evidence that these medications may lower the risk of future TIA.

Some experts recommend in some cases the use of medications which even more effectively prevent blood clotting. These medications are heparin and warfarin. Both are effective in prevention of blood clot formation in other medical problems. Their use is somewhat controversial in transient ischemic attacks and depends on the situation. Surgery is sometimes considered when atherosclerosis with narrowing and blockage of the carotid artery in the neck is discovered. This atherosclerosis in the arteries of the neck is thought to be a common cause of transient ischemic attack. In certain cases an operation is possible in an attempt to remove the blockage from the artery. The operation is called carotid endarterectomy.

Possible treatments for stroke include close observation, usually in hospital, to be sure no complications happen. Complications include worsening of the stroke, difficulty swallowing or breathing, pneumonia, and other medical problems. Evaluation for underlying causes of the stroke and control and removal of risk factors for atherosclerosis is usually planned. Medications such as aspirin and dipyridamole may be used in an effort to decrease further episodes. Other specific medical treatments depend on the cause of the stroke and the individual situation. Your physician may ask that you see a neurologist, a physician specializing in diseases of the brain and nervous system.

Treatment of stroke also includes vigorous attempts at returning as much as possible to the previous level of function. This can be very frustrating to patient and physician. Treatment of weakness in the hand, arm, foot, and leg is greatly helped by a physical therapist and occupational therapist who will teach exercises and help improve activity and ability to carry out daily activities. Physical therapy is extremely important after a stroke and may make a difference in how independent the patient becomes. It is important that the exercises are performed properly twice daily as soon after the stroke as it is medically safe to begin.

It is difficult to predict immediately after a stroke just how much recovery of function may happen. Especially at first, the outlook may appear poor. It may take up to one year to see how much return of muscle strength may finally happen. During this time patient and physician may become discouraged and frustrated.

It is very important to continue attempts at exercise and rehabilitation. If a regular exercise program is not continued then some improvement which is possible may not happen. A physiatrist, who is a physician specializing in rehabilitation medicine, may be very effective in managing the exercise and rehabilitation after a stroke.

■ SWALLOWING DIFFICULTY (DYSPHAGIA)

Dysphagia, or difficulty swallowing, is a common problem. It may reflect any number of causes from nerve or blood vessel disease or, on occasion, a tumor. There may be difficulty swallowing with the sensation that liquids are being returned to the nose, or dropping down into the lungs with a coughing and choking sensation. On occasion, a sensation of blockage in the passage of food may occur and this may arise from a tumor in the throat or esophagus, or from an out-pouching of the throat or esophagus (diverticulum). It may be a result of a stroke, when it happens along with other symptoms such as vision abnormalities, hoarseness, or speech difficulties. It is important to know that stress can produce a process called globus pharyngus which gives the symptom of the proverbial "knot in the throat" that temporarily disappears with swallowing only to return. Whatever the cause, it is imperative to have this symptom evaluated by the internist (Gastroenterologist) or otolaryngologist (ENT specialist). Fluoroscopy with swallowing, and possibly even endoscopy whereby an instrument is passed down the throat through the mouth may be used for an accurate diagnosis.

■ SYSTEMIC LUPUS ERYTHEMATOSUS

Systemic Lupus Erythematosus (SLE or Lupus) is one form of arthritis which is more common in women, especially in the ages 20–40. It may also happen in older men and women. The most common problem is arthritis, but many other problems can happen including fever, rash (rash on the face may appear like a butterfly across the cheeks), severe fatigue, and internal organ disease. Lupus can cause disease in the kidneys, brain, heart, lungs, and other organs. This disease may be confused with many other diseases and may be very difficult to diagnose. This delay in diagnosis may add to the frustration these persons feel from the disease alone.

In addition to discussion and examination, blood tests are helpful in making the diagnosis of Lupus. About 95 percent of patients have a positive blood test for antinuclear antibody (ANA). Other blood tests may also be helpful. Although at times difficult, the overall combination of problems usually allows proper diagnosis.

Treatment includes moist heat and exercises for the joints to keep them flexible and to strengthen muscles. Proper rest is important for the fatigue. Anti-inflammatory medications may help control the joint pain and stiffness and fatigue. At times other medications including prednisone or another cortisone derivative may be needed to control the disease when it attacks the kidneys, brain, heart or other organs.

Systemic lupus erythematosus in years past had a high mortality. Better methods with earlier diagnosis and more effective treatment have changed that situation. Most patients may now expect to live a near normal lifetime with careful treatment and follow up by their physician.

■ SWELLING (EDEMA)

Excess fluid in an area of the body is called edema. This can happen in any area from many different causes. The swelling may be painful but often there is no pain at all. It is easily seen as swelling in the feet and legs. Light pressure by a finger may leave a temporary depression. Edema in the feet and legs is commonly caused by a decrease in the flow of blood in the veins of the legs. Normally the arteries carry the blood toward the feet from the heart. And normally the veins and the lymph vessels return the blood and tissue fluid from the feet back towards the heart. Often the arteries supply the blood to the feet normally, but the veins or lymph vessels do not as effectively return the blood and tissue fluid toward the heart. Then excess fluid may accumulate in the feet and lower legs.

Some common causes in this situation are abnormal veins such as varicose veins (dilated veins). When veins become dilated they don't work as well to return the blood up the legs toward the heart. Edema commonly occurs which is worse when standing or sitting with the feet hanging, such as on a long auto or airline trip. This swelling is usually improved by elevating the feet and legs and by wearing supportive or elastic hose. See other discussion of varicose veins on page 19.

Other common causes of swelling or edema in the legs and feet include blockage of the veins in the legs by blood clots as in thrombophlebitis (blood clots in the veins of the legs or pelvis).

Edema in the feet and legs is also common in heart failure, especially chronic heart failure as a result of the higher pressures in the veins of the legs. Edema is common if the lymph vessels become blocked by any cause. This can happen in an injury or an infection after damage to the lymph vessels. Treatment includes treatment of the underlying cause.

Edema can happen in any area of the body. The swelling after an insect bite, an ankle sprain or an allergic reaction are examples of edema. Swelling and edema may happen after lymph vessels are removed in surgery. For example, it is common to see edema in the arm on the same side after some types of breast surgery if lymph vessels are removed. Edema can occur in the brain after certain injuries and illnesses. Some forms of edema are not serious and disappear, such as after a mild injury. Other forms of edema in the brain may be life-threatening.

The cause of the edema and the effects of the swelling are important. For example, edema and swelling from an insect bite may not be serious in some areas of the body. If the bite happens around the mouth or throat the swelling might cause difficulty breathing.

If you notice any persistent swelling which cannot be easily explained (especially if the swelling is painful or comes on suddenly) you should contact your physician.

■ TEMPORAL ARTERITIS

Temporal arteritis is a disease caused by inflammation in the arteries, and takes its name from problems in the temporal arteries on the side of the head just in front of the ear. This disease affects mainly those persons over 60, and almost always over 50. Headache is common and usually prominent. There may be pain in the muscles of the jaws when chewing food. There may also be fever, weight loss and fatigue. There may be pain and stiffness in the shoulders and upper arms and in the thighs and hips just as in polymyalgia rheumatica (see page 212). If untreated, there may be sudden loss of vision in an eye or other complications.

There may be tenderness on palpation over the temples at the sides of the head. There may be tenderness over the upper arms, shoulders, and thighs. There may be little else to see.

After discussion and examination, blood tests usually show a very abnormal sedimentation rate just as in polymyalgia rheumatica. In fact, at times it seems both diseases are present. A simple biopsy of a temporal artery under local anesthesia may provide the diagnosis.

Treatment requires prednisone or other cortisone derivative. The dose is higher than in polymyalgia, but there is usually a very quick improvement over a few days. Then the dose of prednisone is gradually decreased over a period of many months as long as improvement continues. If treated early there are usually no permanent complications of temporal arteritis but the prednisone required may cause some side effects of its own. Many of these may be able to be controlled or managed with your physician's help.

▪ TENDONITIS

Tendonitis refers to inflammation of the tendon, which attaches a muscle to a bone. The inflammation may cause pain, swelling, warmth and difficulty using the nearby joint. An example is "tennis elbow" which is tendonitis of the muscle that attaches at the elbow. It is common in persons who make the movements which are done in tennis, as well as baseball, golf, and other activities. Other areas which may be bothered by tendonitis are the shoulder and the Achilles tendon near the heel.

Tendonitis may cause severe pain with use of the muscle or nearby joint. Treatment may include the use of rest, moist heat or ice, a careful exercise program, and at times anti-inflammatory medications. Local injections for relief of pain and occasionally surgery may be necessary in some cases. Avoidance of repetitive use of the muscle may help prevent a recurrence of the problem.

▪ THYROID DISEASE

The thyroid gland in the neck produces thyroid hormone which regulates many of the body's activities. If the level of thyroid hormone is abnormally high or low significant illness may happen. The two most common problems are low level of thyroid hormone (hypothyroidism) and abnormally high levels of thyroid hormone (hyperthyroidism). Both problems cause illness and may have a number of different causes. Most causes are quite treatable after proper diagnosis.

In hypothyroidism the level of thyroid hormone is low. Feelings usually come on very gradually over months or years. The most common feelings are those of fatigue, lethargy, low pitched or hoarse voice, constipation, and dry skin. Weight gain is common. These feelings are inconvenient, but if left untreated then hypothyroidism can become more serious and eventually be life-threatening, especially if other illnesses happen.

Tests which will be planned after discussion and examination include blood tests which measure the level of thyroid hormone present. Other tests will be needed to be sure no other problems are present.

Treatment consists of a medication which provides thyroid hormone to return the level to normal. Usually there is improvement in energy and the above changes gradually resolve over months. Follow up is needed to be sure that levels remain normal.

In overactive production of thyroid hormone, the level of hormone is elevated (hyperthyroidism). There are a number of causes of this problem which are treatable after proper diagnosis. Feelings usually begin gradually. The problem is more common in women. Nervousness, rapid heart beat, weight loss, and fatigue are the most common early feelings. Weakness, feeling more uncomfortable in warm environments, restlessness, difficulty sleeping and shortness of breath may occur.

The diagnosis is often suspected by the combination of findings, especially in a female. Blood tests can confirm the problem by measuring the level of thyroid hormone in the blood. Other tests will be sure that no other diseases are present.

Treatment is available depending on the cause of the hyperthyroidism. Your physician can guide the treatment which is effective in controlling the symptoms and correcting or controlling the underlying cause.

Enlargement of the thyroid gland can happen with the overall level of thyroid hormone remaining normal, becoming low, or becoming higher than normal.

If you notice enlargement of the neck or notice a lump in the neck then one of the possibilities is enlargement of the thyroid gland. Enlargement of the thyroid gland is referred to as goiter. There are a large number of causes which require further medical evaluation. Many causes of goiter are not serious but may require treatment.

Some causes may be more serious, including cancer, but may be very treatable if detected early. If you notice any suspicious changes then check with your physician.

■ BLOOD IN URINE (HEMATURIA)

Hematuria refers to blood in the urine. Blood may be visible in the urine or may only be seen when the urine is examined under the microscope. There may be no pain or there may be discomfort depending on the cause of the blood in the urine. One of the most frequent causes is urinary tract infections.

The treatment for urinary tract infection usually includes antibiotic therapy along with increased fluid intake.

Other causes of blood in the urine include stones in the kidney, bladder, or ureter (discussed on page 201). Kidney diseases, bladder diseases including cancer, prostate diseases and other medical problems can result in blood in the urine. The importance of finding blood in the urine is that it can serve as a way to detect problems in the urinary tract at an early stage before other symptoms or signs are present. In all cases, whether the blood is present in large or small amounts, a thorough evaluation is needed.

Tests which may be ordered include IVP (intravenous pyelogram), urine and blood tests, and examination of the bladder. Most persons who have evaluations for blood in the urine are not found to have cancer. But this can be an easy way to detect serious underlying problems at a time when they are more easily and effectively treated.

■ URINARY TRACT INFECTION

Urinary tract infection is most commonly caused by bacteria. Urine is normally sterile. When infection is present in the urine there may be no feelings or signs or infection may be severe and life-threatening. Infections in the urinary tract are most dangerous when there is blockage of urine flow in the presence of infection. Most infections are very effectively treated with antibiotics. In some cases surgery may also be needed to remove an obstruction or stone.

Bladder infections are more common in women because the female urethra is one to two inches in length and more easily infected by bacteria in the genital area. The most common symptoms are frequency and pain on urination. Blood may appear in the urine.

Urinary tract infections in men are often caused by blockage or obstruction to urinary flow. This most commonly happens because of prostate disease. As men advance in age there is often enlargement of the prostate called benign prostatic enlargement (benign prostatic hyperplasia). There may be difficulty in starting or stopping the urinary stream. Eventually blockage of urine flow from the bladder may be more complete. Because the urine is not completely cleared from the urinary system bacteria are not washed away as well and may result in infection and obstruction to urine flow. In these cases antibiotics and surgery may be needed to prevent more severe infection and kidney damage.

Tests which may be ordered include test of the urine for infection, blood test and x-rays. The IVP (intravenous pyelogram) is a test in which a dye is injected into a vein and x-rays are taken of the kidneys, ureters and bladder. These x-rays greatly help to find diseases of the kidney and ureters.

Other tests may include cystoscopy in which a light is inserted into the bladder for direct examination by the urologist. A sonogram of the bladder may be planned which is a painless test to evaluate tissues in the pelvis and kidney areas.

The computed tomographic (CT) scan is helpful to show causes of obstruction and other diseases which may contribute to infection. Magnetic resonance imaging (MRI) may help in some cases to show other problems not detected by CT scan.

Specific treatment of the urinary tract infection as well as any underlying problem is important. Your physician or urologist will guide you in your own situation.

■ WEIGHT LOSS

Weight loss which is unplanned is often alarming, especially in the mature adult over age 50. Most persons who notice unexplained weight loss are most concerned about the possibility of cancer. It is true that many forms of cancer may cause weight loss, but many other medical problems may also account for the weight loss. In mature adults weight loss is common with age as discussed on page 13. This happens with no other underlying disease present. It seems that there is simply an "adjustment" to a lower body weight.

When weight loss is unexplained then medical evaluation is needed. Weight loss can be a sign of a large number of medical problems, many serious and some which can be ignored.

After a discussion and examination, it is usually necessary to plan some laboratory studies including blood tests, x-rays and other studies. The number of tests needed will be greatly determined by the information which your physician has obtained from discussion and physical examination. The more information available, the more likely an early diagnosis with fewer tests will be possible. The basic problem is to be sure no other serious medical problem is present. It is necessary that there be satisfaction that no other serious disease is present.

Treatment depends on the cause of the weight loss. Treatment of the underlying problem and correction of nutrition and eating habits are important.

■ WHEEZING

Wheezing refers to noises made during breathing that are usually high-pitched and come from the bronchial tubes. Wheezing can be caused by many problems which result in narrowing of the bronchial tubes. You may have a cough or feel short of breath from the underlying problem. Wheezing may come and go or can be continuous. Wheezing is not normal and should be evaluated by your physician.

Breathing may be more rapid or more difficult or there may be no noticeable changes. You should not wait for visible changes to see your physician.

After a discussion your physician may order a chest x-ray, blood tests, tests of lung function and other tests depending on the most likely causes of the wheezing.

Treatment will vary depending on the specific cause of the wheezing. Some common causes of wheezing include asthma, acute and chronic bronchitis, emphysema. Other bronchial and lung diseases and heart disease can cause wheezing as well.

CHAPTER 8

The Mature Years: A Time for Growth

One of the most important changes in recent years is the change in perception towards retirement and the mature years. With the increasing number of mature adults each year along with medical advances allowing for a greater, healthier lifespan, many people are coming to see this as a positive time rather than a negative time. Suggestions for entering retirement years with an attitude of expectation follow:

1. One outstanding feature about mature living during the retirement years is that your time is your own! You are now absolutely free to do whatever you would like. There are far fewer restraints. No more punching time clocks or writing weekly expense reports or going to the office even if you don't feel like it. You don't even have to eat at a specific time to accommodate growing children. During the retirement years, the choice every day is *yours* to fill. There is no one to make you do *anything*. You can do what *you* want to when you want to. For many mature adults, this new freedom is frightening. To see retirement as a time of self-discovery, you must take advantage of this freedom and *dream*. That's right . . . dream. Dream about everything you have ever wanted to do or to become. NOW is your opportunity to put into action some of these dreams.

◼ LEARN NEW HOBBIES AND SKILLS

Many people talk about the many hobbies that they have "always wanted to do if they could just find the time." Well, now's the time to do them. Find out about hobby groups, activity groups, interest groups in your area. The local adult education program available through your public schools offers a plethora of programs where you can learn new skills. You can have the pleasure, joy, and fulfillment of realizing dreams that have long been put on the back burner. You can make new friends and expand your horizons.

If you enjoy activity, you can get involved in groups that like to *do* things together. There are many travel clubs; these are not necessarily high priced. There are places within easy driving distance that you have never seen or never been to. Again, now is the time to see them. There are exercise groups, dance clubs like square dancing and ballroom dancing, hiking groups, and walking groups. The limits are only those you self-impose, or those imposed by a physical problem. In the earlier portions of this book, we addressed physical problems and how to limit them.

◼ RENEW FAMILY TIES

One of the most neglected areas of modern life is the connections of the nuclear family. With life being as busy as it is these days, and with families spread out in different locations, the old "homestead" family living is almost extinct. These mature years afford an excellent opportunity for renewing and restoring family ties. This is the generation of the active grandparent. It is *most* important that these relationships continue to be established and strengthened. The mature years are one of the best times for strengthening, renewing, rekindling, and perhaps re-establishing family ties.

◼ CONTINUE YOUR EDUCATION

Another possibility for the mature adult is that of taking advantage of educational opportunities. An amazing array of opportunities are available today. Many community colleges and universities allow mature adults to audit classes at no cost or at very little cost. Wouldn't this be a great time to get some of that college education you always wished you had? Or to expand your horizons and your mind? And it doesn't have to be at the college or university level, because as mentioned earlier, almost every community today has programs of adult education with a broad spectrum of offerings and opportunities. Check these out and take advantage of your schedule to "go back to school."

■ VOLUNTEER TO SERVE OTHERS

This next suggestion might not seem at first as exciting or as appealing as some of the others, but it is vitally important. The mature years are a time when men and women are *"liberated to serve."* The worst thing that mature adults can do is to center only on themselves. This is an outstanding time to get involved with others—a time when you are "liberated to serve." One of the ways to do this is to teach or volunteer in the local school system. Other ways to get involved include your community hospital, religious groups, charitable organizations, day care centers, or other nonprofit groups. Many mature adults have taken it upon themselves to share their skills and knowledge with others. There are never enough volunteers to meet the current needs. Look around, see what interests you, and get involved!

■ JOIN LOCAL ORGANIZATIONS

Another positive opportunity is the chance to get involved in local organizations that you never had time for before. Civic clubs, conservation clubs, garden clubs, political organizations, and many others are out there waiting for you to get involved. Try a lot of things. You might not like one group, so feel free at this time of life to move on to another group until the right interest meets your needs.

Let's review some of the positive opportunities that present themselves to the mature adult:

1. Take advantage of your time—it is your own!
2. Learn new hobbies, skills, activities.
3. Take advantage of travel opportunities.
4. Renew ties with family and friends.
5. Expand your horizons with educational opportunities.
6. Share your skills and talents with others.
7. Get involved in local clubs, groups, and organizations.

The worst thing a mature adult can do during these years is to do nothing or not make adjustments as times change. Harry, a 68-year-old military colonel, loved to fish and retired to a place in Florida where the fishing was supposed to be outstanding. Many other avid fishermen also heard about this place and soon there were many people living there, and the fishing deteriorated. Rather than find a new interest since he couldn't fish, Harry literally *stopped living*. In his mind, he decided if he couldn't fish that he just wouldn't do anything, and he didn't. Harry just vegetated for the next 5 years making life miserable for himself, his wife, and his friends. This is most tragic, but it is reality and happens to many people—especially retired men.

With the amazing opportunities available, mature adults can make these years the best of their lives. Be positive—make it happen. Only *you* can do it.

■ COPING WITH STRESS

As mentioned previously, the leading killers in our society are coronary heart disease, cancer, stroke, diabetes, and atherosclerosis. While researchers are searching for cures for these diseases, we know that there are steps that can be taken to eliminate our risks for getting the disease. One of the most important risk factors in each category for each disease, is eliminating stress.

Let's look at some of the most common symptoms of stress:

1. Tightness in the chest
2. Rapid or pounding heartbeat
3. Difficulty in sleeping or sleeping too much
4. Irritability
5. Lack of concentration
6. Upset stomach
7. Sweaty palms
8. Lethargy
9. Clenched jaws

For many mature adults, stress has become a way of life. For some adults who are living alone with health problems or on a fixed income, this stress results in even more symptoms. Often mature adults feel bleak about the outlook of their lives as they dwell on their worries. And, quite honestly, many of life's stressors are out of our control.

But no matter what is causing the stress, everyone has the ability to make choices about dealing with it. While quite often you can't make the problem or stress disappear, you can react to it in positive ways which can greatly reduce its affect on your emotional and physical being.

1. Get plenty of physical exercise. Excess hormones produced from stressful situations can be worked out of the system by exercise. Whether your program includes aerobics, walking, riding on a stationary bicycle, or gardening, this exercise can enable you to release the tension built up inside. The fresh air and sunshine of outdoor activity assist in supplying extra oxygen and vitamin D that your body needs.

2. Set aside time to relax and meditate. This means time to be alone, whether it is walking to the mailbox each day or watching the sunset in the evening or listening to a favorite tape collection. This relaxation can enable you to relax those muscles that are held so tight during stressful moments.

3. Get proper nutrition and plenty of sleep. Take care of yourself especially during stressful times. Getting enough sleep and eating the proper foods allow the body to repair itself from being torn down by the stressful event. If you can't sleep, lie in bed in a restful position and allow your body a chance to renew.

4. Eliminate stressful situations. Many of the factors creating stress in your life can be eliminated or avoided. First, you need to accept what cannot be changed, then you need to change what you can. Avoid stressful situations when you feel at your breaking point such as heavy traffic, loud noises, too many people, making hasty decisions. Try to make necessary changes in things that you have control over such as living arrangements, time management, hobbies, and other. Accept those stresses that you cannot solve and learn to live with them such as illness in the family, a limited budget, problems with adult children.

5. Seek help before you feel burdened. For many people, religion, church groups, or support groups can help in relieving stress as caring and a sense of objectivity is felt. If you feel you have handled your stress the best you can and still feel overwhelmed, seek professional counseling from your religious leader, a doctor, or other trained professional.

6. Use your network of friends. Often close friends or family members can assist you in stressful times as they listen without giving unsolicited advice. Leaning on your friends, family, or children can be a great asset during these moments.

7. Maintain your regular routine. This is especially important if you are undergoing a life crisis such as the death of a spouse or child. It is vital that you continue to get up each morning, get dressed, and plan your days just as you did previously in order not to fall into a depression.

Our bodies and minds were meant to handle stress. Because stress is a reality in life, it is vital to manage it so you can use your energy on activities that bring pleasure and meaning to your world.

■ DEALING WITH DEPRESSION

Although people tend to be social creatures, we have an amazing habit of focusing in on self. This simple act of introspection, as useful as it is, can also be one of our worst enemies. In fact, it is the leading contributor to a malady that affects millions of mature adults today; it is known under the wide umbrella of the most common mental illness—*depression.*

Depression generally occurs when negative thoughts compound upon themselves and get so rooted into the subconscious that we cannot break out of the cycle of negativism and self-pity. If left untreated, depression can last for months or even years leading to feelings of helplessness and, at worst, suicide.

Depression is very debilitating and ruins life for millions of people. As many as 10 million Americans experience depression in their lives. This figure extends to as many as 13 to 20 percent of the total population in the United States having depression at any given time. Twice as many women undergo depression as men.

Depression is a very complicated problem, and not as easy to deal with as many suspect. Many times depression can stem from a biochemical imbalance or it may be a symptom of an underlying ailment. Quite often, professional medical help is needed to maintain, control, and cure depression with medication and therapy. There are many excellent prescription drugs and many medical protocols that can assist greatly if this is the case.

However, there are some practical choices that the mature adult can make to stop the cycle of mild depression before it gets out of control and becomes a major problem. This is not to confuse mild depression with the sadness or grief that is experienced with the loss of a loved one. Of course, those feelings of sadness are normal and to be expected.

Symptoms of depression include:

- Disturbances in sleep patterns
- Loss of interest in usual activities
- Weight loss or gain (more than 5 percent of body weight)
- Fatigue
- Impaired thinking
- Thoughts of dying or suicide
- Irritable moods for extended periods

Of course many people may have one or more of these symptoms at one time or another. The problem occurs when these problems and symptoms begin to occur on a daily basis for a period of at least two weeks. If you or someone you know has these symptoms on a regular basis, you must seek professional help for a diagnosis and follow your physician's advice in taking medication and/or receiving therapy to alleviate the problem.

■ LEARN TO LIVE ONE DAY AT A TIME

Many situations of mild depression are caused because people "borrow trouble from tomorrow." They forget that we have enough to deal with today, and we don't need to borrow troubles from tomorrow. On the flip side of that, many people also "borrow trouble from the past." All of us have had to deal with some form of heartache or despair in our lives, but we keep bringing those things up from the past. One of the first and best things we can do to break the cycle of depression is not to borrow trouble from either yesterday or tomorrow. The adage "live one day at a time" is an excellent cure for depression if you can channel your thoughts into this positive way of thinking. Some researchers have found it is helpful to replace negative thoughts and worries with positive thoughts of the moment. For example, instead of dwelling on a past conflict with a friend or family member, think only of an event that is occurring at the moment such as baking that pie, or going shopping or playing golf or visiting with the new grandbaby. Every time the negative thought comes to mind, replace it immediately with a positive thought. You will be surprised at how quickly you can train your mind to eliminate thoughts about past situations or future worries which you have no control over.

No one but you can eliminate these negative thoughts for you. You must take control of these thoughts and replace them with positive thinking that will enable you to move forward in your life.

Sometimes depression is caused because we "create" or "invent" troubles that aren't real. We forget that we have enough to deal with in life just as it is, without creating problems that don't even exist. Wouldn't it be great if we could be content to deal with what is already before us without adding additional difficulties?

Write down on paper all of your worries, real and imaginary. Save this piece of paper and look at it one month, three months, and six months from this date. Chances are none or very few of these worries actually became a reality. Most of the worries and depressed thoughts people have are fabricated in the mind. Don't let your mind be an inventor, especially when it comes to negative thoughts.

It helps greatly to be realistic about things and to accept them as they are. Sometimes the perspective of an outside observer is helpful. This can be a close personal friend, a doctor, a minister, a counselor, a therapist, or any person who will just listen and help us to sort things out without giving a lot of unsolicited advice.

Talk out your real problems. Find a friend who will listen and get these troubles off your chest. You will feel a sense of freedom as you discuss openly any concerns that are truly bothering you. Then, do something positive instead of continuing to dwell on these real problems.

■ TIPS FOR COPING WITH DEPRESSION

Here are some other useful tips for dealing with depression as developed by the American Cancer Society.

1. Be careful about focusing in on yourself too much. Be aware of "self-talk." There are too many people who can *never* sing that old song "Nobody Knows the Trouble I've Seen" because they talk about them all of the time, and everyone knows about their troubles. The cycle of depression begins when we get too focused on ourselves and our own problems. We must catch ourselves at being too self-centered in our conversation.

2. Concentrate on dropping certain words from your vocabulary—words like "can't" and "should." A famous musician told of a
piano teacher he had as a child:

> I had a piano teacher who frequently admonished me about us-
> ing the word "can't." He shared this during an interview after a sym-
> phony performance. Whenever I was in a lesson and said: "I *can't* do
> it," she would always stop and correct me and say, "You *can* . . . but
> you won't." Those words of sage advice have always stayed with me.

Eliminate words like "can't" and "should" from your vocabulary
and substitute words like "can" or "want to."

3. Another corollary is that we should get involved in something larger than ourselves. Reaching out to help others is a great way
to get our minds off of ourselves, and it greatly reduces the beginnings
of depression that are caused by brooding, moping, or too much self-
introspection.

4. Learn to say "no" once in awhile also. There is a difference
between doing things for others and having others take advantage of
you. Sometimes we get depressed because we feel trapped in a situation
we can't get out of or we feel we've lost control. We have to know that
it is OK to say "no" once in awhile if we feel that unreasonable and
undue pressures are being placed upon us, even by those we love. We
are in control!

5. Talk things out. There is no better therapy than this. Bot-
tling up all your worries and fears only builds up tension. We often
lose perspective of things when we keep them inside. As the cycle of
introspection, brooding, moping, and self-pity gets started, we often
lose sight of the original problem. Talking things out once in awhile
with someone can give us a new perspective, and it also stops the cycle.

6. Learn your limits—know your limitations. Pace yourself. We
often push ourselves beyond our limit. We need to know how far
we can go, and stop before we get tired.

7. Sometimes we are our own worst enemies in that we feel
that we always have to "win." Some people feel that they must always
be right and must always win every argument. Evaluate your own
personality and realize that you don't have to always win. Often the
amount of energy used in winning an argument is not worth it. In
fact, it sometimes helps to let the other person win once in awhile.
Often depression is caused by our own need for superiority and our
need always to be right. When we don't win, we feel let down and

rejected. This can create a great deal of stress, tension, and anger that inevitably leads to depression. Give in once in awhile.

8. Not enough can be said about the need for exercise in our life. Physical activity is perhaps the most valuable method of letting off steam and releasing tension, frustration, and boredom. Walking is a popular form of exercise for people of all ages. Sitting around brooding and feeling sorry for ourselves only contributes to the cycle of depression. For those who are unable to go out-of-doors or are limited in mobility, many communities offer light exercise classes in community centers and even in malls before hours. Aquatic exercises are offered at low costs at local YMCAs. Check out some of these things, and get busy. Active people are seldom depressed people.

9. Develop leisure activities that you enjoy whether it's a hobby, a project, or joining a club. Time spent with others is often therapeutic. When people spend too much time in solitude, depression, sickness, and disease are the inevitable results. Get out! Get involved! Stop sitting around!

10. Don't let life overwhelm you. Take one concern at a time. Figure out what is most important in your life, and take care of it. Establish priorities. The old adage "divide and conquer" is a valuable rule for us to follow when life seems so overwhelming. When we get overwhelmed, we can sometimes fall victim to a condition known as "analysis paralysis." That is a condition where we can't get going because we have so many options before us creating overwhelming feelings. Look at the following ways to work through overwhelming times:

- Develop problem-solving skills. First, identify the problem and write it down so it's clear in your mind. Get a good idea of just what the problem is so that it is clear in your mind.
- List your options, list the possibilities, both pro and con. Make lists.
- Choose a plan.
- List the steps to carry it out.
- Give yourself a deadline and act.

Many times just having a plan and some options helps to break the cycle of depression.

11. Even though we have heard it over and over again, we still must be reminded of the importance of "focusing on the positive." For instance, if we suffer a setback, we should immediately concentrate on our achievements. Focus on what you have accomplished in

your life, on your talents and gifts, on your successes—accentuate the positive.

12. Much depression is caused by lack of proper nutrition and lack of adequate sleep and rest. We must take care that we eat properly, regularly, and that we do not allow ourselves to get overtired. Many of us have problems eating alone, and so this is an opportunity for us to invite others over, or become part of organizations that have regular meals together. Many civic and church organizations meet regularly for meals together. Take the initiative and be responsible for proper nutrition and proper rest to prevent the cycle of depression from getting started. Look at the wealth of nutritional advice in Chapters 7-9. Follow these guidelines for improving your overall nutrition and mental outlook.

13. Finally, try to find some humor, joy, and pleasure at least once a day. Look at the newspaper cartoons or even the situation comedies on TV. Make it a point to have at least one good laugh a day, and you'll be well on your way to battling depression.

The guidelines and suggestions that we have included in this chapter have been found to be practical and helpful. We recognize, however, that dealing with depression is no easy matter, and often it is *not* possible for someone to "snap out of it." Many times it takes skilled professional guidance to assist in dealing with depression, and we certainly recognize that fact. However, we also recognize that by following a few easy steps and guidelines, we can establish patterns of living and thinking that will greatly diminish the possibility and the risks of mild depression.

■ PLANNING FOR ILLNESS AND DEATH

Inevitably, despite all of our best efforts, there will come the time when we must face the crisis of illness or even death. Most people are surprised when sudden illness or death occurs. Many people seem to live their lives as if they are going to live and be healthy forever, and do not give the slightest thought to the possibility that they may become ill or dependent some day. It is often this shock that causes most of the problems initially when serious illness occurs. They "can't believe" it happened to them. The simple reality of life is that all of us are going to die. Therefore, one of the best things that we can do is to literally "prepare" for it. Talk about it with your spouse or with your family and have a plan of action *written down* to use when this occurs to you. This is not macabre; this is realism and will go a long way toward making those you love have an easier time accepting your death.

There are too many people who find themselves in a problem or a crisis, without ever having given the slightest consideration to such possibilities. The best advice you can have is to "be prepared." Live the best—hope for the best—expect the best, but also be sensible enough to anticipate and plan for the worst case scenario, if it should occur. Many mature adults find great comfort and strength in religious organizations or in a power greater than humankind. Knowing that death and illness is inevitable, look for that strength that will enable you to cope when it happens in your life.

Too many cases have shown the persons in crisis situations are often too distraught to think clearly and rationally. We recommend a well thought out plan of action during times of crises to be helpful.

■ CREATING A CRISIS PLAN

Talk about it. It may sound simple, but the first and best thing we can do is to talk about the situation whether it be fear of an illness, loneliness, or death itself. Checklist 9 is for you to use in formulating your crisis plan. Fill in the appropriate blanks and keep this for referral should you need it.

Many questions need to be asked, and a plan of action developed. Write your personal crisis plan down on paper for other family members to have and tell them where this plan is. Often older adults are faced with unexpected crisis and have not even considered that illness or death could occur. This creates incredible confusion and lack of rational thinking combined with the shock of the event. Sometimes the stresses of the current moment so greatly enhanced the crisis, that it made it almost impossible to make some very important decisions. Sometimes clear thinking does not go along with times of crisis, so a well thought out plan of action is of most value, especially if it is written down. While you can't anticipate everything, your crisis plan is a beginning for coping with the mature years in a responsible way, and at least you will have some clear picture about what to do should the unforeseen happen.

Discuss all of the possibilities and options that will occur should unexpected illness or death happen in your family, and develop a plan of action. Write down your plan with your family members and spouse.

Place this crisis plan in an important file along with other papers such as your will, insurance records, and important papers. Then, enjoy your life knowing that you are prepared should unexpected crisis occur.

■ LEARN TO CARE

Caring is vital in dealing with crisis and it is important to learn how to care. Many of us do not have the skills or understanding it takes to be a caring person. When a loved one is found to have a terminal illness or unexpectedly dies, we often feel inadequate in dealing with that person or other family members.

If someone you care about is diagnosed with a serious illness or is experiencing another life crisis, it is important to always face the truth. If you begin to hedge with the person or tell untruths, you will find barriers between you and communication becomes stifled. When communication halts, the person in crisis remains puzzled and usually begins to fear the worst about their situation.

Do not set limits with the terminally ill person. The sick person is tempted to want to know "when will this happen" or "when will that happen" or "how much time do I have," and so on. This temptation must be resisted, and the person must be encouraged to maintain the hopeful attitude of taking one day at a time.

Be a listener with sensitivity when dealing with people in crisis. We must subjugate our own fears and anxieties in order to listen to what the person is really saying and feeling, and then respond to his needs accordingly. Be alert to the specific needs the person may have. He may be hesitant to ask, so be alert and sensitive to what you perceive may be needed whether it be placing your arm on his; calling a religious counselor, hospital chaplain, or pastor; or getting other family members into the room.

Never allow a person in crisis to feel abandoned. Always assure him that you will be there for him, and make arrangements that care is provided should you have to leave to take care of your own life.

Don't try to give medical advice. That is the duty of the doctors and nurses, and even though we may feel we know what's best from our own experiences, we must not tread on their ground. This sometimes causes tension, anxiety, bitterness, and confusion. Let the doctors do their job!

Most important, always hold out hope, but not false hope. Even a little hope is better than no hope at all, but again, be honest, open, caring, and loving. Continue to be positive. Not all illnesses are terminal, and most patients who are ill or undergo surgery recover to live active and useful lives for many years. Don't give in to the temptation to feel sorry for yourself, and strive to maintain a totally bright and positive outlook.

As mentioned earlier, however, the best plan is to have a plan. Be sure that you do not postpone making these arrangements before it is too late.

Here are some other suggestions that may be helpful in your planning.

1. Be aware of what kind of nursing care is available in your area. For instance, persons recovering from strokes and major surgery may not be able to stay in hospital for the entire length of recovery, and are not able to be cared for at home either. What do you do? Have a plan of action in case something like this happens. Visit the different facilities in your area, see what they offer. Find out the costs, services, and so on.

2. Find out what kind of social services are available for mature adults in your community. Though the demand for these services is increasing in many areas, it is amazing that many services go unused because people simply do not know to seek out the assistance. Anticipate the worst case scenario, and plan for it. At least have an idea of what is around. See Chapter 12 for a complete listing of services available in most communities and through the U.S. government.

3. Among the most neglected items among mature adults today is the will and the pre-arranged funeral. See Chapter 9 for important information in planning for death and/or death of a spouse. So many times there is additional trauma during an unexpected death simply because there was no will and the funeral arrangements were not pre-arranged. People are so reluctant to face up to these inevitable things, that many times they live to regret their postponing these decisions. There are many organizations in every community that can give assistance in this pre-planning. AARP, Social Security, funeral homes, and local county aging offices have tremendous amounts of available information and assistance in this type of pre-planning.

Remember, make these plans and arrangements as early as possible. The testimonies of those who did are sufficient evidence for the importance of this planning. You only have to experience *one* situation where proper planning was not done, to convince you of the importance of this.

■ FACING DEATH

It is never easy to accept death. When a loved one has died, we may often feel angry, confused, or emotionally numb. We may not know how to express our feelings of loss, or how to say goodbye to the person who has died. But we need to work through these feelings because, again, they are inevitable. They will occur to all of us. Accepting and realizing this is one big step on the road to facing up to and dealing with death.

It is a sad thing that death in our society has become so sterile, and institutionalized, and so far removed from the course of everyday events. It wasn't that long ago when most people died at home, and families were involved in the process all along. But with medical advances in recent years, then with life-saving procedures and equipment ever on the increase, the death process has become increasingly an institutional one. What this has tended to do is to shelter and to hide the reality of death from many people. It is not uncommon, for instance, for persons to be well into their adult years, and still have *never* attended a funeral or seen a dead person. Our culture seems adamant on trying to hide the fact that death is a part of life, therefore, we hide the sick and the infirm away in hospitals and nursing homes, and when death comes it usually occurs behind closed doors with no close relatives around. Sometimes even the rituals of funerals seem to shelter us from the reality of death, and we are content to want to sweep the whole issue of death under the rug. This is foolish, of course, but how do we deal with the whole issue of death? Here are some suggestions:

1. Face the reality. Accept it. Get it straight in your mind that death is going to come into your life. Acknowledge the fact that you will one day be leaving this life for the next. Therefore, live the very best you can now, in order that you will have no regrets when the end comes. Don't put off until tomorrow what you ought to be doing today. This life is incredibly short, so don't let it pass you by.

2. In order to avoid feelings of guilt later, do what you should be doing now. Do for one another now what you may wish you had done later. In other words, have NO regrets and guilt when a loved one passes away. Don't neglect doing those little things. Ask yourself: "What if 'so and so' were to die today? What would I have wished I had done? What regrets might I have?" If there are any, go ahead and take care of them now, not when it is too late. Think of some nice

little things that the other person would really appreciate, and start doing them.

3. Don't let your life revolve around just one person. Although that might sound a bit insensitive, cruel, and uncaring, there is a great deal of truth to that statement. Too many couples have lived with their complete and total life revolving around each other only. They had no outside friends, no outside activities, no outside interests. Though this may sound beautiful and romantic, it is very impractical, because it is always devastating to the remaining spouse when the other becomes ill or dies. Develop a full life *now*. Have some outside interests, friends, and activities. This doesn't take anything away from your relationship, but it *does* expand your horizons and give you a fuller and broader approach to life. It also allows you to get on with life later. Though you may be deeply in love and the very best and most intimate of friends, do not let your life be completely absorbed in any one person. It isn't right to you or the other person, and it isn't fair.

4. After death or loss of a spouse or loved one, get on with your life. Again, this requires a realistic and wholesome outlook, and some anticipation of this time coming. But, if you are realistic in your approach, you will not allow your mourning and grief to be excessive or to drag out for long periods of time. Often professional counseling may be considered if you find yourself not responding to the world each day and living in grief or in the past.

5. Funerals are a positive force in the grieving process and can be helpful. As stated earlier, death is not easy to face or to accept for anyone. But funerals can help us to work through our feelings. A funeral is a ritual that can help focus our emotions and bring meaning to the experience of death. Rituals link us with the past and the future. We have rituals for graduations and marriages, and we need a ritual for this most important passage of life. The funeral serves as a means to commemorate the deceased, but just as importantly, it helps the survivors to heal emotionally. When someone we love dies, we experience the pain of grief. But even though it hurts, grief is not something to avoid. This is most important . . . we *must not* avoid grief. Grief, in fact, is a part of the healing process that allows us to separate ourselves from the deceased person and to go on with our lives.

Funerals give persons a ritual "permission" to express their feelings of sadness and loss. Funerals also stimulate persons to begin talking about the deceased, one of the first steps toward accepting death. In fact, people who do not attend the funeral of a loved one because they want to deny the death may suffer from unresolved grief several months later. To resolve their grief, people need to accept the reality of death not only on an intellectual level but on an emotional level also. It is for this reason that funerals in our culture are usually preceded by an open-casket visitation period. Research has found that the viewing of the deceased person helps you to accept the death of that person. It helps with grieving because it shows that there is no return to this life and it is final. Funeral directors and clergy persons are helpful in guiding persons through this time, but again the real key to coping with this time is *pre-planning*.

6. The time of the death of a loved one can also be a time of opportunity for the remaining spouse. Sometimes, the spouse has had the burden of care and the responsibility for the person, and with the person passing on, they are often freed up for new dimensions of living and new opportunities never explored before. Sometimes the windfalls of judicious planning such as life insurance policies, also provide an economic stability and freedom that allows greater flexibility in life. These are some things that need not be overlooked in the process of carrying on with life. We hear it over and over again, where we say that the person who has passed away would not want the remaining spouse just to sit around and do nothing all the time, and this is true. There is certainly nothing to be gained from unnecessarily prolonging the grief process. This is not insensitive and uncaring. Often the burden of many years of constantly caring for an invalid or ill person ends with death. Opportunities can now be taken for the caregiver to enrich his own life. Be aware of these needs in your practical planning for your life.

Death is an unavoidable reality, but with faith, proper living, proper planning, and proper attitudes, it need not be a crippling experience. With the proper outlook, death is a life change that we can live with and through, and continue to make those discoveries of self that are vital.

■ GOAL SETTING FOR THE MATURE ADULT

Goals are vital for any human being. They help turn your hopes and dreams into purpose and reality. Without specific goals, the mature adult has no guidelines for living. These goals become especially important when stumbling blocks such as depression or illness enter into one's life. You can evaluate your personal goals periodically and determine if your life is on track. You can also make changes as you look over your life goals and adjust these accordingly.

Let's look at the following steps that can assist you in making personal goals that will enable you to live a positive and fulfilled retirement life.

1. Ask yourself: What would I like to see happen in my life?

Again, remember to dream! Brainstorm. Picture your life a year from now, five years from now. What do you visualize? Perhaps a trip abroad, a move to a new dwelling, or a new hobby is in your dream. Maybe your dream is more specific such as overcoming a lengthy illness or recovering from a recent surgery.

Write down these dreams in a notebook for these can become reality in the near future.

2. Ask yourself: What would it take to make these dreams into realities?

Now take the same notebook and list on paper the planning steps that could help meet these problems or dreams head on. Perhaps you would need to meet some friends for travel companions to take that special trip. Maybe you would need to send away for brochures of various cities if you are planning to relocate. Perhaps a visit to the hobby store or taking classes through the city's recreational department would allow that new hobby to become a reality.

If your vision is to get well from a lengthy illness, perhaps a complete health plan including proper nutrition, exercise, medication, and positive thinking can be the specific steps you need to take. Or if you want to recover from a recent surgery, the steps might include following the physician's orders with therapy, bedrest, and proper nutrition.

Dreams only can become a reality when you make it a point to take the necessary steps to fulfill the dreams.

3. Review your goals weekly.

Just like the goals you set when you were younger gave meaning to your life as you prepared for the first career, raising a family, or buying a home, the goals you set as a mature adult also give meaning to your retirement years.

Reviewing your goals weekly helps you to see how well you are following your dream. Your personal faith in yourself will be strengthened and your outlook on life will become brighter as you find success in meeting your goals.

4. Evaluate your goals as your personal needs change. Once you take that big trip abroad or make that move to a new city, you need

to adjust your goals. The new goals need not be extravagant. Rather, you must aim to produce balanced growth in all aspects of your life as a mature adult—emotional, spiritual, physical, and social. New goals might be set which include:

Making a new friend
Losing five pounds
Starting an exercise program
Writing your biography
Helping a neighbor
Volunteering at the hospital
Planting a garden
Traveling around the world
Visiting a grandchild
Looking up old friends
Researching your family genealogy
Learning a new hobby
Starting a part-time career
Redecorating your home

The success of your life as a mature adult depends on how seriously you address YOUR personal needs through goal-setting and how well you follow through in attempting to meet these goals.

■ FORESIGHT IS THE KEY

Human life brings with it many challenges and changes and opportunities. These occur at every stage in the process. However, the challenges and changes and opportunities that face us during the mature years require planning, insight, and wisdom if they are to be met and dealt with in a positive and helpful way. The mature years can be exciting years if faced with realism and foresight. The unrealistic fantasy touted by such movies as *Cocoon* and *Cocoon II* is just that . . . fantasy. Life *does* go on . . . we *do* grow older . . . and we *must* deal realistically with the dangers and pitfalls, as well as the opportunities that the mature years bring. So rather than looking for the "fountain of youth," let us look inside and find our true potential in the mature years as we strive to be the best we can.

CHAPTER 9

Planning for Financial Changes

Financial pressures during the mature years can have a tremendous impact on our physical and emotional well-being. While this stage in life should be filled with the realization of dreams including retirement, travel, hobbies, different careers, new friends, volunteering, and reading those many books collecting on the shelf, often these dreams are not fulfilled because of lack of money.

Financial planning should be an ongoing process throughout a lifetime. Yet, many mature adults exist on a budget that is far less than the amount they lived on as younger and middle-aged adults. The added stress of paying unexpected bills, increasing inflation, and health care costs during retirement can ultimately take its toll on health and well-being resulting in depression and stress-related illness.

But this period of life can be an exciting time if the right financial choices have been made. Sudden health problems may begin to surface and many older adults find they are unable to work as hard in later years. So careful financial planning *before* retirement is mandatory to ensure comfortable and worryfree living *after* retirement.

■ WHAT IS FINANCIAL PLANNING?

Financial planning for retirement involves much more than merely figuring out where your income source will be. If you are still young, financial planning for your mature years will allow you to make choices including pension plans, IRAs, investments, health and life insurance, savings, property ownership, and more. If you are nearing retirement age, financial planning may assist you in using your securities to best advantage by drawing interest income from investments or living within your means. Let's begin to put together the plan that will lead up to a comfortable retirement including consideration of your total net worth, health insurance plans, and available assistance for special health needs.

It has been estimated that an amount needed for retirement years should be from 50 to 80 percent of your normal working income. The following actions can move you toward this retirement income goal.

Before Age 50

1. Review all insurance as your children approach independence.
2. Direct your investments toward long-term growth.
3. Increase retirement savings and develop an estate plan.
4. Review and update your will.

During the 50s

1. Maximize savings as family expenses decline.
2. Consider tax and inflation hedges in investments.
3. Begin to lay out your specific retirement program.
4. Update your will.
5. Contact Social Security to check their records of your earnings and obtain all pamphlets needed for retirement planning.

During the 60s

1. Restructure your investments for income and safety of principal.
2. Pay off all debts before retirement.
3. Review insurance needs, update will, and finalize estate plans.

■ RETIREMENT PLANNING

There are many different factors to consider when planning for retirement years. Consider Checklist 7 and mentally fill in the appropriate blanks to begin your complete financial plan.

CHECKLIST 7
RETIREMENT PLANNING

1. What retirement benefits are available from my employer?

2. How does Social Security, Medicare, and government programs fit into my financial plans?

3. Have I thoroughly reviewed the insurance coverage for retirement years along with pre-Medicare and Medicare benefits? What will this coverage include?

4. Do I want to shift my investments to more conservative income producing investments? If so, which ones?

5. Should I consider trading my present dwelling for smaller quarters such as a condominium or apartment to lessen the burden of upkeep on a home? If so, how much is my present dwelling worth?

6. Do I need the equity out of my present home to meet my retirement goals?

7. Do I plan to supplement my retirement income with part-time work or projects which would add monetary assistance? If so, which ones and how much money do I anticipate making?

■ APPROACHING RETIREMENT YEARS WITH CONFIDENCE

Perhaps you had a difficult time answering these pertinent questions. Let's look at a few ways to approach retirement years allowing for maximum freedom and financial security. Begin by taking inventory of your assets, expenses, and income. As the dollar amount unfolds, you will be able to determine your present financial position which will offer ways to use your assets for an acceptable retirement. Remember, the peace of mind you have during the mature years with adequate financial security can and does affect your mental and physical health. We emphasize that this is only an example of retirement planning, but it can force you to take inventory of your assets and start putting the finishing touches on your retirement plan. Careful discussion with your financial advisor should take place before making any changes in the use of your assets. (Your financial advisor may be your financial planner, accountant, insurance agent, attorney, broker, etc.)

Calculating Your Net Worth

As you begin taking inventory of your assets, you need to calculate your net worth. Net worth is your assets (what you own) less your liabilities (what you owe).

You will want to preserve your net worth and have it grow faster than inflation until the time you retire. Your net worth will be your primary source of income to cover your retirement expenses.

To help you comprehend the use of net worth, we have used an example of one couple planning for retirement in two years. After filling out the suggested forms, they have established their net worth to be $175,000. Let's see how they determined this amount (Figure 7).

■ EXPENSE ADJUSTMENTS FOR RETIREMENT

Once you determine your net worth, you can work out your expenses and determine the adjustments that can be made for your retirement.

Fill in an expense worksheet like the one in Figure 8 showing in column A your current expenses on an ongoing basis. Column B will show the effect retirement will have on each current expense and should give you some idea of the income required to cover retirement expenses. Recognize that you are dealing with today's expenses and at retirement you will have to consider inflation. In

FIGURE 7
Net Worth Form A for Sample Couple
(Current Year)

	Amount ($)
Assets—What You Own	
1. Retirement plan including IRA	13,500
2. Total bank funds (cash)	1,500
3. Other income investments (bonds, CDs, etc.)	15,000
4. Common stocks including mutual funds	26,500
5. Real estate investment (market value) equity	8,000
6. Other investments (business interest, collectibles, other)	5,000
7. Net value of business	0
8. Market value of home	90,000
9. Life insurance cash value	8,000
10. Personal property, i.e., furniture, jewelry	30,000
11. Automobiles(s)	8,000
12. Miscellaneous (money owned to you, security deposits, etc.)	0
13. *Total Assets*	$205,500
What You Owe—Liabilities	
14. Balance on mortgage(s)	(25,000)
15. Taxes due	0
16. Auto loans	(3,500)
17. Other loans	(1,000)
18. Monthly bills (credit cards) & other short-term obligations	(1,000)
19. *Total Liabilities*	(30,500)
(Total 14 thru 18)	158
Net Worth (13) less (19)	$175,000

doing this, you can make the adjustments necessary to cover those inflated expenses.

Look at the following categories that must be considered as you figure out your retirement expenses.

1. *Housing.* Consider your housing status at retirement. If you stay in your present dwelling and your payments are reduced or paid off, what changes can be expected? You may want to consider moving into smaller quarters such as a condominium or apartment or renting instead of purchasing a dwelling. If your present home was sold, you could invest the equity and in addition reduce your expenses for each

FIGURE 8
Expenses Form for Sample Couple

Expenses	Current Year Column A	Changes Column B	Retirement (A less B) Column C
1. Housing mortgage, taxes, utilities, electricity, water, gas & oil	$ 8,500	($ 1,700)*	$ 6,800
2. Food incl. entertaining at home	6,500	(1,500)	5,000
3. Transportation, car payments, repairs, fuel	4,000	(1,500)	2,500
4. Clothing & linens	2,000	(500)	1,500
5. Insurance—property, auto, health, life	2,000	(0)	2,000
6. Medical & dental	1,500	1,000+	2,500
7. Contributions & gifts	1,500	(1,000)	500
8. Repayment of loans, credit cards	1,000	(1,000)	0
9. Recreation—entertainment, vacations, sports events, hobbies	3,000	(1,000)	2,000
10. Miscellaneous expenses	2,000	(1,500)	500
11. Savings & retirement IRAs, company plan, investments, other	3,800	(2,500)	1,300
12. Taxes (local, state, federal)	8,000	(7,200)	800
13. Totals	$43,800	($18,400)	$25,400

*Parentheses denotes a negative change, that is, subtract $1,700.

category of housing such as upkeep, insurance, taxes, utilities, and so on. Place an estimate for this reduction. *Caution:* Be sure you qualify for the over 55 tax break on the sale of your house.

2. *Food.* Will you be reducing your entertaining costs and work-related meals away from home? Extra time might be used in shopping for sale items or using coupons. Enter any reduction on this line.

3. *Transportation.* If you have two cars, it is worth considering cutting back to one during retirement years. With only one car, you can realize a reduction in car payment, maintenance, insurance, and taxes. Commuting expense will be eliminated. You may consider doing car repairs or washing your car rather than paying others to do this. Enter a carefully thought-out reduction here.

4. *Clothing.* You should realize a reduction in clothing costs eliminating work suits, uniforms, dress, and possibly some cleaning bills. Enter a reduction here.

5. *Insurance.* Be discriminating as you search for senior citizen's discounts on your homeowners' and automobile insurance. Advise your agent as to the reduction in miles used for commuting to work. Consider a smaller car for less insurance and fuel cost. If you move into smaller quarters, the homeowners' insurance should be less. Be sure to review other insurance coverage with your agent to see if any change would result in lower costs. Enter any reductions here.

6. *Medical and Dental—Out of Pocket.* With careful planning, you should review the following possible choices:

- A Medicare participating physician
- A PPO or HMO
- Medigap coverage
- Nursing home coverage
- Prescription costs
- Effect of Medicare Catastrophic Protection

These choices should minimize the out-of-pocket costs for medical and dental bills. A slight increase in costs might be expected here.

7. *Contributions.* Work contributions will end at retirement as well as reductions in contributions based on your income. Volunteering for religious organizations and other charities can make up for the smaller contributions. Enter a reduction here.

8. *Loans and Credit Cards.* Loans should be repaid at retirement and credit card use should drop considering the absence of work-related expenses and less entertainment costs. Enter a reduction here.

9. *Recreation.* With more free time, your choices for entertainment and vacations should favor those establishments catering to and offering senior citizen's discounts. Careful planning should permit a slight reduction here.

10. *Miscellaneous Expenses.* Consider reducing those items not required for retirement. Painting and maintenance of a home, remodeling, and so on. Reduce subscriptions for magazines. Enter a reduction here.

11. *Savings and Retirement.* This item should have an important reduction as we begin to use those assets instead of storing them except to cover inflation. Enter a reduction here.

12. *Taxes.* Withholding and Social Security taxes should be minimal. A sizable reduction should be possible here.

13. *Total Columns A, B, & C.* Column C is the amount retirement expenses are estimated to be.

Various studies have indicated that careful retirement planning can adjust retirement expenses to a range of 50 to 80 percent of preretirement levels depending on your goals. For the couple used in our example, the retirement expenses would require an annual income of $25,400 (58% of preretirement income).

■ INCOME ADJUSTMENTS FOR RETIREMENT

To complete this example of how to accomplish your retirement goal, our sample couple chose to liquidate all assets except for one automobile, most furniture, and certain personal items.

The proceeds from the liquidated assets can now be invested to produce retirement income. The net worth of $175,000 less $30,000 personal property and $8000 for the automobile would leave $137,000 to invest at 8 percent and would return $10,960 per year. In addition to this income, a retirement of $2400 per year from employment plus an amount of $15,084 per year from Social Security (from the table), would then give a total income of $28,444. When we apply the projected expenses of $25,400 (which includes $1300 savings) to the balance of $3044, this would give us a total amount of $4344 additional spendable income, savings, or to cover inflation. Once you go through the formula and figure out your total retirement finances, you can then make necessary adjustments that might be required to accomplish retirement goals. Whether this year or in 10 years, you only need to update the totals filled in on these pages using your current information and adjusting for inflation to project the retirement results. The objective is to have retirement income to equal retirement expenses. This approach would permit retirement without touching the principal resulting in long-term income at this level. Use of the principal should be avoided as it would deplete the fund and reduce future income. The retirement income can be supplemented by part-time work or other income-producing projects, such as hobbies.

Figure 9 shows how our sample couple plans to fund their retirement. Now is the time to begin your plan. The earlier you lay out your plan, the more time you will have to make adjustments and fine tune your retirement.

After working through the example, look at your projected income and retirement goals. You should have a clear picture of an acceptable retirement plan if you decide to take early retirement or retire tomorrow.

FIGURE 9
Retirement Income Form for Sample Couple

	This Year	Year _____
Investment fund $ 137,000 at 8% %	10,960	_____
Retirement income from employment	2,400	_____
Income from Social Security (from chart)	15,084	_____
Other income	0	_____
Net income	28,444	_____
Projected expenses at retirement	(25,400)	(_____)
Additional spendable income	3,044	_____
Plus savings	1,300	_____
Savings (inflation fighter)	4,344	_____

Personal Income Form

	This Year	Year _____
Investment fund $_____ at ____%	_____	_____
Retirement income from employment	_____	_____
Income from Social Security (Use Tables 44; 45)	_____	_____
Other income	_____	_____
Potential retirement income	_____	_____
Net income	_____	_____
Projected expenses at retirement	(_____)	(_____)
Additional spendable income	_____	_____
Savings (inflation fighter)	_____	_____

■ PROJECTING FOR THE FUTURE

How can you alter this minimum goal and put into action those changes that can improve your retirement benefits? Once you clearly define the goal, you can take advantage of the benefits that only time can offer such as:

- Increase your personal savings, IRA, work retirement plan, or Keogh
- Reconsider your investment strategy to obtain a good return that protects the capital of the retirement fund
- Join those organizations such as AARP or professional organizations that can offer continued planning and information
- Take advantage of senior citizen's discounts (most start at age 55) and receive discounts from restaurants, motels, prescriptions (AARP and several drug store chains)
- Review your insurance coverage, your financial statements, investment strategy, and check funds on record at Social Security every one to three years prior to the retirement date.

Make financial adjustments early and let your retirement goals unfold according to your plan. As you are assessing your financial net worth and expenses for retirement, it is also time for you to plan your activities. An interest or hobby started today should be under way *before* the retirement date arrives if you are counting on income from this to subsidize your retirement fund. Your time will need the same careful planning and preparation as your finances. Retirees can experience almost any activity to supplement income such as woodworking and handcrafts, collecting at flea markets and garage sales for resale, working part-time, and more. But it is important to start now preparing a plan that will have these profit-making activities under way before that retirement day arrives.

The mature years can be a rewarding, fulfilled time in anyone's life. Remember the following formula for retirement success:

1. Lay out the plan including formulating your net worth, knowing your expenses, and having adequate health insurance policies.
2. Fulfill the plan by sticking to your retirement budget.
3. Enjoy the riches of retirement by filling your days with meaningful activities that give you a sense of well-being.

■ COST OF HEALTH MAINTENANCE

The period of retirement can be the most costly period for your health maintenance. For the past 10 years, escalating health care costs have become a national problem and have exceeded inflation in most years. One major health care provider lost 66 million dollars in 1987 with an additional 40 million dollar loss in 1988. We see insurance premiums increasing faster during the late 1980s than for any previous period. Increases up to 25 percent for group coverage and up to 40 percent for Medicare supplements have occurred in many states in the past year. For the person looking forward to retirement years, these facts can create uncertainties.

If you are considering early retirement, be certain that the benefits you took for granted during employment will continue without change, and know the exact cost of the policy. The problem of changing health care policies is becoming more difficult and caution must be taken during this period. If you choose early retirement and must switch coverage, be sure that any pre-existing condition is covered. If not, evaluate the cost to cover the condition until the waiting period is over. Use *caution* and do not assume that health care coverage as an employee will be the same after retirement. Discuss this openly with your insurance agent to be sure you have selected the best option that will give you peace of mind and security of benefits.

Under the Consolidated Omnibus Budget Reconciliation Act of 1986 (COBRA), the terminated employee has certain rights for continued coverage for the employee and/or dependents under group insurance if he or she pays the employer's cost plus 2 percent for the coverage. There is a statutory limit on how long this coverage may be available, but do not hesitate to look into this act if you have concern on extending your insurance coverage.

■ MEDIGAP COVERAGE

If you have group coverage upon reaching Medicare age you should explore the possibility of converting the group coverage to a Medicare (Medigap) supplemental coverage.

The cost for the Medigap supplemental coverage will be much less and by continuing with the same company providing the group coverage, it might offer more benefits than purchasing from some other source. Also, by continuing with your group carrier, you won't have a problem with pre-existing conditions. Again, there is still a strong caution in switching coverage even after Medicare because a pre-existing condition may not be covered with a new carrier. Blue Cross-Blue Shield, AARP, and many other top insurance companies offer excellent Medicare (Medigap) supplemental coverage.

■ SOCIAL SECURITY—IT WORKS FOR YOU

Call your Social Security office and request the free brochures available for retirement planning. Social Security has been paying benefits for almost 50 years. It is a federal government program for you and your family members when you retire, become severely disabled, or die. It is designed to replace part of the income you normally would receive from employment. It is a base to build on, now and in the future, with other insurance and investments, such as private pensions, personal savings, and other assets.

Social Security does not operate like a bank. Rather, it is a pipeline. Revenues collected from today's workers flow into one end of the pipeline and come out the other end in the form of benefits for today's beneficiaries—a sort of pact between generations.

You and your employer each pay an equal share of Social Security (FICA) taxes. If you are self-employed, you pay taxes for retirement, survivors, disability, and hospital insurance at a rate twice the employee rate.

Table 43 shows the Social Security tax rate effective for January 1988 through 1989 and for 1990 and later.

TABLE 43
Tax Rate for You and Your Employer (each)

Percent of covered earnings

Years	For Retirement Survivors, and Disability Insurance	Hospital Insurance	Employee and Employer Rate	Total
1988–89	6.06	1.45	7.51	15.02
1990 and later	6.20	1.45	7.65	15.30

Tax Rate for Self-Employed People

Percent of covered earnings

Years	For Retirement, Survivors, and Disability Insurance	Hospital Insurance	Total
1988–89	12.12	2.90	15.02
1990 and later	12.40	2.90	15.30

■ TAX CREDITS

Self-employed people will receive a credit against the self-employment Social Security tax rate of 2.0 percent of self-employment income for 1986–1989.

After 1989, this credit will be replaced with deductions designed to treat the self-employed in much the same manner as employees and employers are treated for Social Security and income tax purposes under the present law.

■ WHAT YOU RECEIVE FOR YOUR SOCIAL SECURITY TAXES

You receive two things for your Social Security taxes—monthly benefits and insurance protection. Most people understand the concept of Social Security, but few know the extent of the monthly benefits they will eventually receive when they retire. Many people do not realize that while they are working, they have insurance protection for themselves and their families should they die or become severely disabled.

This is a very important part of Social Security. Everyone wants to be relatively healthy until they retire, but we know that death and disability can and do strike people of all ages. In fact, it is estimated that about 3 out of every 10 people who start working today will die or become severely disabled before reaching normal retirement age.

■ QUALIFYING FOR SOCIAL SECURITY BENEFITS

The normal retirement age is 65 years; that is the age when you are eligible for full retirement benefits. But you can start receiving reduced benefits as early as age 62, and your spouse can receive them at the same age. If your child is under 16 or disabled, is receiving Social Security benefits and is in your care, you can receive spouse's benefits regardless of your age.

The amount of your benefit depends on how old you are, when you apply, and your lifetime earnings on which you paid Social Security taxes. Other earnings and other types of income are not used to figure your Social Security benefit. You can call the Social Security local office in your city and ask officials to estimate your personal benefits. The higher your average earnings in your lifetime, the higher your benefit rate will be from Social Security when you retire. (See Tables 44 and 45.)

Medicare Benefits

Part of the FICA taxes withheld from your pay are for Medicare. When you become 65, you will be eligible for Medicare even if you keep on working at your employment. Also, you are eligible for Medicare if you have been receiving disability benefits for 2 years or have permanent kidney failure.

Are You Eligible for Social Security Benefits?

For a worker and family to receive monthly cash benefits, the workers must have earnings credits for a certain amount of work under Social Security. Almost every kind of job, as well as self-employment, fits in this category.

In 1987, you earn one credit for each $460 of earnings you have during the year, up to a maximum of four credits for $1840 or more of earnings. This includes gross wages paid to you and net self-employment income. In 1988, these dollar figures will be $470 for one credit and $1880 for four credits, and they will increase automatically in future years as average wages increase.

When a person has a certain amount of credits, we say that he or she is "fully insured" and can receive monthly benefits at retirement age.

No one can be fully insured with less than 6 credits (1 1/2 years of work), and a person who has credit for 10 years of work can be sure that he or she will be fully insured for life for retirement or survivors' benefits. Having enough credits to be insured means that certain kinds of Social Security benefits can be paid—it does *not* determine the amount (Table 46).

How the Disability Program Works

Social Security provides basic protection against the loss of family income due to the disability of a major income earner. Part of the Social Security taxes paid by employees, their employers, and self-employed people is used to finance the program.

Under Social Security, the definition of disability is related to the ability to work. A person is considered disabled when he or she

TABLE 44

Approximate Monthly Survivors Benefits if the Worker Dies in 1988 and had Steady Earnings

Worker's Age	Worker's Family	Deceased Worker's Earnings in 1987						
		$10,000	$15,000	$20,000	$25,000	$30,000	$35,000	$43,800 or more
25	Spouse and 1 child[1]	$668	$864	$1,060	$1,226	$1,318	$1,410	$1,572
	Spouse and 2 children[2]	717	1,073	1,263	1,432	1,539	1,646	1,834
	1 child only	334	432	530	613	659	705	786
	Spouse at age 60[3]	318	412	505	584	628	672	749
35	Spouse and 1 child[1]	662	856	1,048	1,220	1,310	1,400	1,516
	Spouse and 2 children[2]	706	1,056	1,252	1,424	1,529	1,635	1,769
	1 child only	331	428	524	610	655	700	758
	Spouse at age 60[3]	316	408	500	581	624	667	722
45	Spouse and 1 child[1]	662	854	1,046	1,216	1,286	1,332	1,384
	Spouse and 2 children[2]	705	1,054	1,251	1,420	1,502	1,555	1,616
	1 child only	331	427	523	608	643	666	692
	Spouse at age 60[3]	315	407	499	579	613	635	660
55	Spouse and 1 child[1]	660	866	1,046	1,194	1,242	1,272	1,306
	Spouse and 2 children[2]	703	1,067	1,250	1,395	1,451	1,485	1,524
	1 child only	330	433	523	597	621	636	653
	Spouse at age 60[3]	315	412	498	569	592	606	622
65	Spouse and 1 child[1]	638	824	1,012	1,152	1,194	1,224	1,256
	Spouse and 2 children[2]	682	1,021	1,206	1,345	1,395	1,429	1,468
	1 child only	319	412	506	576	597	612	628
	Spouse at age 60[3]	304	393	482	549	570	583	599

[1] Amounts shown also equal the benefits paid to two children, if no parent survives or surviving parent has substantial earnings.

[2] Equals the maximum family benefit.

[3] Amounts payable in 1988. Spouses turning 60 in the future would receive higher benefits.

Note: The accuracy of these estimates depends on the pattern of the worker's earnings in prior years. See text for details. To use the table, find the age and earnings closest to your age and earnings in 1987.

267

TABLE 45
Approximate Monthly Retirement Benefits if
Worker Retires at Normal Retirement Age with Steady Lifetime Earnings

Worker's Age in 1988	Worker's Family	Retired Worker's Earnings in 1987						
		$10,000	$15,000	$20,000	$25,000	$30,000	$35,000	$43,800 or more
25	Retired worker only	$618	$801	$983	$1,129	$1,214	$1,300	$1,471
	Worker and spouse[1]	927	1,201	1,474	1,693	1,821	1,950	2,206
35	Retired worker only	572	740	908	1,045	1,123	1,203	1,358
	Worker and spouse[1]	858	1,110	1,362	1,567	1,684	1,804	2,037
45	Retired worker only	523	677	831	958	1,030	1,092	1,201
	Worker and spouse[1]	784	1,015	1,246	1,437	1,545	1,638	1,801
55	Retired worker only	475	614	754	862	910	946	1,003
	Worker and spouse[1]	712	921	1,131	1,293	1,365	1,419	1,504
65	Retired worker only	425	550	675	768	797	816	838
	Worker and spouse[1]	637	825	1,012	1,152	1,195	1,224	1,257

[1]Spouse is assumed to be the same age as the worker. Spouse may qualify for a higher retirement benefit based on his or her own work record.

Note: The accuracy of these estimates depends on the pattern of the worker's actual past earnings, and on his or her earnings in the future. See text for details. To use the table, find your age and the figure closest to your earnings in 1987. These figures will give you an estimate of your retirement benefits at various ages.

TABLE 46

The following chart shows how much credit for work covered by Social Security you need to be fully insured.

For Workers Reaching Age 62 in	Years of Credit Needed
1984	8 1/4
1985	8 1/2
1986	8 3/4
1987	9
1988	9 1/4
1989	9 1/2
1990	9 3/4
1991 or later	10

Note: You are fully insured if you have one credit for each year after 1950 up to the year you reach 62, become disabled, or die. In counting the years after 1950, a person born in 1930 or later would omit years before 22.

has a severe physical or mental impairment or combination of impairments that prevents him or her from working for a year or more or that is expected to result in death. The work does not necessarily have to be the kind of work done before disability—it can be any gainful work found in the national economy. This definition requires total disability and is somewhat stricter than the definition of some other programs that may pay benefits in cases of partial disability.

Once people are on the disability rolls, benefits continue as long as they remain medically disabled and are not engaging in substantial gainful activity. Their cases are periodically reviewed to see if they are still disabled. But benefits will stop only if they have medically improved and are able to perform substantial gainful activity. To help those who attempt to return to work, a number of special provisions permit them to receive payments while testing their ability to work. In addition, Medicare coverage is available to people who have been entitled to disability benefits for 24 months or who have kidney disease requiring regular dialysis or a kidney transplant (Table 47).

Who Receives Disability Payments

You may qualify for disability benefits as a worker under 65 (workers 65 and over may qualify for retirement benefits). Certain members of

TABLE 47
Approximate Monthly Disability Benefits if the
Worker Becomes Disabled in 1988 and Had Steady Earnings

Worker's Age	Worker's Family	Disabled Worker's Earnings in 1987						
		$10,000	$15,000	$20,000	$25,000	$30,000	$35,000	$43,800 or more
25	Disabled worker only	$459	$595	$731	$837	$900	$964	$1,076
	Disabled worker, spouse, and child[1]	689	894	1,098	1,256	1,351	1,447	1,615
35	Disabled worker only	449	579	710	824	885	941	1,005
	Disabled worker, spouse, and child[1]	674	870	1,066	1,237	1,328	1,413	1,509
45	Disabled worker only	447	578	708	821	869	900	936
	Disabled worker, spouse, and child[1]	672	867	1,063	1,233	1,304	1,351	1,404
55	Disabled worker only	446	577	707	810	842	862	886
	Disabled worker, spouse, and child[1]	670	866	1,061	1,215	1,263	1,294	1,330
64	Disabled worker only	435	562	689	785	813	832	853
	Disabled worker, spouse, and child[1]	653	843	1,304	1,178	1,221	1,248	1,280

[1]Equals the maximum family benefit.

Note: The accuracy of these estimates depends on the pattern of the worker's earnings in prior years. See text for details. To use the table, find the age and earnings closest to your age and earnings in 1987.

your family may also qualify for disability benefits on your work record.

To qualify for Social Security disability benefits, you must have worked long enough and recently enough under Social Security to be insured. (Family members who qualify for benefits on the worker's record do not need credits of their own.) In 1988, you earn one credit of coverage for each $470 in earnings, up to four credits with annual earnings of $1840 or more. The amount of earnings required for these credits increases each year as the general wage levels rise (Table 48).

TABLE 48

The number of years of work credits needed for disability benefits depends on your age when you become disabled.

- Before 24—You need 6 credits in the 3-year period ending when your disability starts.
- 24 through 31—You need credit for having worked half the time between 21 and the time you become disabled.
- 31 or older—You need the amount of credit shown below. Also, you generally must have earned at least 20 credits in the 10 years immediately before you become disabled. You also need to have as many total work credits as you would need for retirement.

Born After 1929, Become Disabled at Age	Born Before 1930, Become Disabled Before 62	Credits You Need
31 through 42		20
44		22
46		24
48		26
50		28
52		30
53		31
54		32
55		33
56		34
57	1986	35
58	1987	36
59	1988	37
60	1989	38
62 or older	1991 or later	40

Exception: If you are disabled by blindness, the required credits may have been earned at any time after 1936; you need no recent credit.

What Conditions Are Disabling?

Medical evidence from your physician or other sources should show how severe your condition is and to what extent it prevents you from working.

The following are examples of conditions that ordinarily are severe enough to be considered disabling. A more detailed list can be found in the Social Security regulations, available at any Social Security office.

- Diseases of the heart, lungs, or blood vessels that have resulted in serious loss of function as shown by appropriate medical evaluation and that produce severe limitations in spite of medical treatment.
- Severe arthritis consisting of recurrent inflammation, pain, swelling, and deformity in major joints so that the ability to get about or use the hands is severely limited.
- Mental illness resulting in marked constriction of activities and interests, deterioration in personal habits or work-related behavior, and seriously impaired ability to get along with other people.
- Brain abnormality resulting in severe loss of judgment, intellect, orientation, or memory.
- Cancer that is progressive and has not been controlled or cured.
- Diseases of the digestive system that result in severe malnutrition, weight loss, weakness, and anemia.
- Disorders that have resulted in the loss of a leg or which have caused it to become useless.
- Loss of major functions of both arms, both legs, or a leg and an arm.
- Serious loss of function of the kidneys.
- Total inability to speak.

If you are a widow or widower, a decision as to whether you are disabled will be based solely on medical evidence. Factors such as age, education, and work experience cannot be considered as they are with disabled workers.

Monthly benefits for a disabled worker or a disabled widow or widower generally start with the sixth full month of disability. If the sixth month is past, the first payment could include some back payments. The amount of monthly disability benefits is based on a worker's lifetime average earnings covered by Social Security. The average monthly benefit for a disabled person early in 1988 was $508, and the average payment to a disabled worker with a family was $919.

■ WHAT IS MEDICARE?

Medicare is a federal health insurance program for people 65 or older, people of any age with permanent kidney failure, and certain disabled people. It is administered by the Health Care Financing Administration (HCFA). Local Social Security offices take applications for Medicare, assist beneficiaries in claiming Medicare payments, and provide information about the program.

Medicare has two parts—hospital insurance and medical insurance. Hospital insurance helps pay for inpatient hospital care and certain follow-up care. Medical insurance helps pay for your doctor's services and many other medical services and items.

Hospital insurance is financed through part of the payroll (FICA) tax that also pays for Social Security. Voluntary medical insurance is financed from the monthly premiums paid by people who have enrolled for it and from general federal revenues.

Who Is Eligible?

You are eligible for Medicare hospital insurance at age 65 if:

- You are entitled to monthly Social Security benefits or railroad retirement benefits
- You have worked long enough to be insured under Social Security or the railroad retirement system
- You have worked long enough in the federal, state, or local government to be insured for Medicare purposes.

You are eligible before age 65 if:

- You have been entitled to Social Security disability benefits for 24 months
- You have worked long enough in government employment and meet the requirements of the Social Security disability program.

Under certain conditions, your spouse, divorced spouse, widow or widower, or dependent parents may be eligible for hospital insurance at age 65. Also, disabled widows, widowers under age 65, disabled surviving divorced spouses under 65, and disabled children 18 or older may be eligible. For more information, contact a Social Security office.

■ GETTING HOSPITAL INSURANCE PROTECTION

Some people have to apply for hospital insurance protection before it can start; for others, hospital insurance protection starts automatically. If you are nearing 65, you do not have to retire to have hospital insurance protection at 65. But if you plan to keep working, you will have to file an application for hospital insurance in order for your protection to begin. You should apply at a Social Security office about 3 months before you reach 65.

If you are receiving Social Security or railroad retirement checks, your hospital insurance protection will start automatically at 65.

If you are a government retiree who is eligible for Medicare on the basis of government employment, you will have to apply for hospital insurance in order for it to begin at 65. Contact a Social Security office about 3 months before your 65th birthday to file your application.

If you aren't eligible for hospital insurance at 65, you can buy it. The basic premium was $234 a month in 1988. To buy hospital insurance, you also have to enroll and pay the monthly premium for medical insurance. If you are an alien, you must be a permanent resident and must reside in the United States for 5 years before you can apply for Medicare. You can apply at any Social Security office.

Who Is Eligible

Almost anyone who is 65 or older or who is eligible for hospital insurance can enroll for Medicare medical insurance. You don't need any Social Security or government work credits to get medical insurance.

Aliens 65 or older who are not eligible for hospital insurance must be permanent residents and must reside in the United States for 5 years before they can enroll in medical insurance.

If you want medical insurance protection, you pay a monthly premium for it. The basic premium was $24.80 a month in 1988.

Some people are automatically enrolled in medical insurance. Others must apply for it. If you are receiving Social Security benefits or retirement benefits under the railroad retirement system, you will be automatically enrolled for medical insurance—unless you say you don't want it—at the same time you become entitled to hospital insurance.

You will have to apply for medical insurance if you:

- Plan to continue working past 65
- Are 65 but aren't eligible for hospital insurance
- Have permanent kidney failure
- Are a disabled widow or widower between 50 and 65 who isn't getting disability benefits
- Are eligible for Medicare on the basis of government employment
- Live in Puerto Rico or outside the United States.

Contact your local Social Security or railroad retirement office for detailed information about medical insurance enrollment.

Medical Insurance Enrollment Period

There is a 7-month initial enrollment period for medical insurance. This period begins 3 months before the month you first become eligible for medical insurance and ends 3 months after that month.

If you enroll during the first 3 months of your enrollment period, your medical insurance protection will start with the month you are eligible. If you enroll during the last 4 months, your protection will start 1 to 3 months after you enroll.

If you don't take medical insurance during your initial enrollment period, you can sign up during a general enrollment period—January 1 through March 31 of each year. But if you enroll during a general enrollment period, your protection won't start until the following July. In addition, your monthly premium will be 10 percent higher than the basic premium for each 12-month period you could have been enrolled but were not.

Special rules apply to workers and their spouses age 65 or older and to disabled people under 65 who have employer group health coverage.

What Medicare Does *Not* Cover

Medicare provides basic protection against the high cost of illness, but it will not pay all of your health care expenses. Some of the services and supplies Medicare cannot pay for are:

- Custodial care, such as help with bathing, eating, and taking medicine
- Dentures and routine dental exams
- Eyeglasses
- Hearing aids, and examinations to prescribe or fit them
- Long-term care (nursing homes)
- Personal comfort items such as a phone or TV in your hospital room
- Routine physical checkups and related tests
- Prescription drugs and patent medicines.

In certain situations, Medicare can help pay for care in qualified Canadian or Mexican hospitals. Otherwise, Medicare cannot pay for hospital or medical services you receive outside the United States (Puerto Rico, Guam, American Samoa, the Virgin Islands, and the Northern Mariana Islands are considered part of the United States).

Many private health insurance companies point out that their policies for people who have Medicare are designed to coordinate their coverage with Medicare. They recommend that their policy holders sign up for Medicare medical insurance to have full protection.

If you have other health insurance, it may not pay for some of the services that are covered by Medicare medical insurance. You should get in touch with your insurer or agent to discuss your health insurance needs in relation to Medicare protection. This is particularly important if you have family members who are covered under your present policy. Also, in planning your health insurance coverage, remember that long-term care (or nursing home care) is not usually covered by Medicare or most private health insurance policies.

If you have health care protection from the Veterans Administration (VA) or under the CHAMPUS or CHAMPVA program, your health benefits may change or end when you become eligible for Medicare. You should contact the VA, the Department of Defense, or a military health benefits advisor for information before you decide not to enroll in Medicare medical insurance.

If you have health care protection from the Indian Health Service, a federal employees' health plan, or a state medical assistance program, the people there can help you to decide whether it is to your advantage to have Medicare medical insurance.

For your own protection, be sure not to cancel any health insurance you now have until the month your Medicare coverage begins.

If you are thinking about buying private insurance to supplement Medicare, make sure it does not simply duplicate your Medicare coverage. If you want help in deciding whether to buy private supplemental insurance, ask at any Social Security office for the pamphlet, *Guide to Health Insurance for People with Medicare.* This free pamphlet describes the various types of supplemental insurance available.

Employers with 20 or more employees are required to offer their workers age 65 or older the same health benefits that are provided to younger employees. They also must offer the spouses age 65 or older of workers of any age the same health benefits given younger employees.

If you are 65 or older and continue working or are the spouse 65 or older of a worker and you accept the employer's health plan, Medicare will be the secondary health insurance payer. If you reject the employer's health plan, Medicare will be the primary health insurance payer. The employer is not allowed to offer you Medicare supplemental coverage if you reject his or her health plan.

Also, if you work after you reach 65 or are a spouse 65 or older and are covered under an employer health plan, you can wait to enroll in Medicare medical insurance during a special enrollment period. You won't have to pay the 10 percent premium surcharge for late enrollment, if you meet certain requirements.

If you are under 65 and disabled, Medicare will be the secondary payer if you choose coverage under your employer's health plan or a family member's employer health plan. This provision applies only to large group health plans. A large group health plan is any plan that covers employees of at least one employer that has at least 100 or more workers. But, you have the same special enrollment period and premium rights under Medicare medical insurance that workers 65 or older have. For more information about these special rules, contact your employer.

If you are under 65, are entitled to Medicare solely on the basis of permanent kidney failure, and have an employer group health plan, Medicare will be the secondary payer for an initial period of up to 12 months. At the end of the 12-month period, Medicare becomes the primary payer.

If you have any questions about Medicare, call your local Social Security office. The phone number is listed in your telephone book under "Social Security Administration" or "U.S. Government."

■ CATASTROPHIC HEALTH INSURANCE

Medicare has been changed to better protect the over 32 million older and disabled beneficiaries from "catastrophic" hospital, doctor, and prescription drug costs. The changes, mandated by the Medicare Catastrophic Coverage Act of 1988 (Public Law 100-360) limits the amount you as a Medicare beneficiary must pay for hospital care, physician services, medical supplies, and outpatient drugs covered by Medicare. It increases home health, skilled nursing facility, and hospice coverage, and adds breast-cancer screening and respite care benefits.

These new and improved benefits will be made available to you automatically if you are a Medicare beneficiary or when you become eligible for the program (Table 49). You are not required to do anything to receive this coverage. If you are enrolled in Part A only and want to enroll in Part B so as to take advantage of all of the benefits, you will be given a chance to do so during the general enrollment period from January 1 through March 31 each year (Table 50).

TABLE 49
Catastrophic Limits
(Medicare Has Been Improved)

Coverage	Old Benefits	New Benefits
Hospital Care— Inpatient	First 60 days in full after $540 deductible for each stay. Days 61–90 must pay $130 daily coinsurance. Days 91–150must pay $260 per day. No coverage after 150 days. Lifetime reserve of 60 free hospital days.	Only one deductible per year regardless of number of admissions $564 deductible 1989; $600 in 1990 with increases thereafter. All costs covered indefinitely.
Doctor's Charges Part B Coverage	After one $75 annual deductible pays 80% of all approved charges.Beneficiary pays 20% copayment plus any amounts above approved charges from nonassigned claims.	Same but with a cap of $1370 per year rising to $1900 in 1993 in copayment and deductible of approved charges.
Nursing Home	Covers up to 100 days per year with copayment of $65 per day after day 20. Must stay 3 days in hospital to qualify. For medical only—no custodial care.	Increased to 150 days per year with 20% copayment after first 8 days. Medical care must be certified by a doctor. No hospital care required. Custodial care not covered.
Prescriptions	No coverage	Start 1990 pays 50% of costs for intravenous drugs

TABLE 49 (Continued)

Coverage	Old Benefits	New Benefits
		used at home ($600 annual deductible) 1991 pays 50% of cost of all prescriptions ($600 annual deductible). 1992 covers 60%, 1993 and thereafter covers 80%.
Home Health Care	21 days per year of skilled nursing limited to 5 visits per week	38-24 hr. days of skilled nursing care must be prescribed by doctor. Additional days may be considered due to medical necessity.
Mental Health Outpatient	$250 per year	Increases to $1100 per year with visits to adjust medication covered under part B, and will not count toward this limit.
Hospice Care	Pays up to $68 per day with limit of 210 days. Home health care will be permitted.	No limit on days. Other benefits unchanged.
Medicaid Changes	Medicaid pays Medicare premiums, copayments and deductibles for beneficiaries with income below 80% of poverty level, which is $6870 per family and $5440 for the individual.	Medicaid pays for Medicare premiums, copayments and deductibles for beneficiaries with income below 100% of poverty level and medical expenses for pregnant women and infants up to one year of age whose income is below the poverty level.
Spouse Income Protection	Most elderly have to spend down to poverty level to qualify for Medicaid.	Medicaid will permit the spouse of the patient who enters the nursing home for long term care to keep $786 of income per month; increasing to $1000 per month by 1993 and may retain $12,000 in liquid assets with home ownership protected by other laws.

TABLE 50
The Cost of "Catastrophic" Coverage
Under Medicare
(Single Beneficiaries in 1989 and 1993)

| Total Income | Annual Surcharge | |
	1989	1993
$5,000–15,000	$ 0	$ 0
$15,000–20,000	78.12	116.52
$20,000–25,000	197.88	250.56
$25,000–30,000	306.96	401.28
$30,000–35,000	370.68	702.00
$35,000–40,000	678.36	1,021.68
$40,000–45,000	800.00*	1,050.00*

Note: All beneficiaries must pay an annual $48 basic premium for the "catastrophic" coverage in 1989 and an estimated $122.40 basic premium in 1993, regardless of income.

*Maximum coverage

Source: Joint Committee on Taxation

■ VETERAN'S BENEFITS

Veteran's benefits are special privileges and services available to qualified ex-servicemen and women and some of their dependents. The services include: institutional care, medication payment, physician services, hospitalization coverage, and certain in-home assistance. The availability of services varies in each region and is dependent on the number of veterans using the services at any one time.

Individuals with service-related injuries/disabilities have first priority. Individuals who served in the armed forces, but whose injuries/disabilities are not service-related come next, in priority rating. If the funds are available, the spouses and/or children of ex-military personnel may be eligible for some services/assistance.

Any veteran can apply for special services through the VA. The application will be appropriately processed and, depending on the disability and the availability of funds for services, the person may be eligible for assistance in acute or long-term care needs.

Many of the VA programs require the person to receive the services at the area VA center or use approved resources to receive maximal benefits available.

The exact services and programs covered vary for each region and over time. It is reasonable to check with the local VA if you think a patient may be entitled to benefits.

■ MEDICAID

Medicaid is a federally funded, state-administered medical insurance program for categorically or medically needy people regardless of age. It is possible for an older person to have *both* insurance policies. Medicare would pay for hospital and physician services and Medicaid would cover medications and routine physical care.

Someone whose income is in the form of a Supplemental Security Income would be considered categorically needy. The amount of the check may range from $10 to $324/month. If applicants meet all other allowable financial reserve requirements, they can apply for Medicaid at the local Department of Social Services. Notification of eligibility may take 45 days. Retroactive coverage is dependent upon multiple factors and cannot be assumed (i.e., nursing homes will generally not take a person who has Medicaid approval pending unless a large deposit is made).

Medically Needy

Someone whose income is in the form of a Social Security payment, but whose medical bills exceed the ability to pay would be considered medically needy. The person may use up to $183/month for living expenses, but all other income must be used for medical purposes. All other reserve requirements must be met and the person must apply at the county Department of Social Services.

Allowable reserve includes:

- $1100 total in checking and savings accounts, bonds, stocks, inherited property, cash value of insurance policies, and other cash assets
- A house and the land it's on (if the person or spouse lives there)
- One vehicle that must be used at least four times a year for medical transport (additional vehicles are valued as part of cash assets)
- Personal burial plot and plot(s) for the immediate family (additional plots are valued as part of the cash assets).

Anyone can apply for Medicaid. Persons who meet both the income limits and the reserve limits are eligible to receive Medicaid benefits for a six-month period.

Medical Equipment

Durable medical equipment (DME)—any reusable appliance or device—can be used for safety or to increase independence. It may be purchased or rented. Much of the appropriate equipment can and should be ordered for a patient before discharge.

Not all equipment is covered by Medicare or Medicaid. Completing all necessary forms will help with the reimbursement. Families may be asked to pay upfront money and fill out Medicare forms for reimbursement process, but doing so won't ensure reimbursement.

Hospice Services

Hospice organizations exist in every state. Call the National Hospice Organization (703) 243-5900 to locate the nearest hospice agency for your patients.

After giving referral information to the organization, patients should expect to wait anywhere from one to three weeks (after discharge) before the hospice organization contacts them. Some agencies have waiting lists and may not be able to see new patients immediately.

In-Home Assistance

In-home services—not including home-health services—are available in most communities. The programs are run by public agencies, nonprofit agencies, and private agencies. Quality of service, reliability, and availability will vary from county to county, town to town, and agency to agency. Some programs originated in social services while others started in health/medical services. These beginnings influence the type and degree of professional supervision, the training of the caregivers, need for physician orders, and reimbursement sources. Some of the programs frequently available are:

- Homeowners
- Personal-care aides
- Chore workers
- Private duty nurses

Eligibility for each of these services is determined by a combination of patient need, reimbursement sources, eligibility, and service availability. If there is adequate money available, most of these services are open to a person with adequate funds. Contact with individual agencies would be needed to determine whether or not the mature adult would be able to get the service in a timely fashion (i.e., short waiting list).

Public Programs

Public programs are a large number of publicly funded community programs for elderly people with limited incomes. These programs are generally operated under the auspices of the local government agencies such as the Department of Social Services (DSS), the Public Health Department (PHD), or Department/Division/Council (Dept/Div/Council) on Aging.

Program quality and size varies greatly from one community to another. It pays to know the local resources before making referrals. The purposes of these programs vary, but in general, they provide services to community dwelling elders. The administrative agencies typically have oversight responsibility for the governmental standards for each program as well as the responsibility for determining eligibility for services and assigning priority to those on waiting lists for services. Programs include:

- Information and Referral. Usually operated by the local Dept/Div/Council on Aging. This service usually offers resources, materials, and information to any/all interested older persons and their families on community programs, housing options, leisure opportunities, and special programs for the elderly.
- Adult Protective Services. Operated by the local DSS. This program is staffed by care workers who investigate any complaints of neglect or abuse of elderly persons. The complaints can be made anonymously. All complaints will be investigated within 48 hours. This service is available to any person, regardless of income. Geriatric specialists should report cases of suspected neglect or abuse to Protective Services for more information.
- Adult Placement Services. Operated by the local DSS. This program uses statewide listings to help families find available beds in nursing homes. Anyone is eligible to use this service.

Some counties have also included the Medicaid-CAP program in this service group. The hospital social workers or discharge planners will also assist in this process if the person is still in the hospital. Medicaid application (if private funds are not being used) will need to be made before placement can occur.

- Fill in the Gaps (FIGS). Operated by the local DSS. This program uses local funds to provide a variety of emergency needs including medications, food, housing, fuel, and other necessities. Help is usually on a one-time-only basis, and funds are very limited. Applications for assistance must be made at the local DSS.

- In-Home Services. These programs can be run by any combination of the public agencies in a county. Each county varies the administration, operation, size, and target population. Services can include chore workers, personal-care aides, and homemakers. Funding varies, but the public funding is usually Title XX, county funds, Medicaid-CAP, community development money (and sometimes private pay). Letters of support from physicians are helpful in shortening waiting lists.

- Food Stamps. Operated by the local DSS. Food stamps are a federally and state-funded program to assist in food purchase for a very low-income person. Recent cuts in this program make its usefulness to the elderly questionable. If they receive an average Social Security check, they will probably be eligible for no more than $10 in stamps a month. Applications must be made every three months, and stamps must be picked up at the post office.

- Rest Homes and Family Care Homes. Subsidies for and regulation of these settings are managed by the local DSS. Eligibility criteria for placement and funding are less stringent than Medicaid requirements, but must be completed prior to placement if public funds are to be used. The availability of these services varies between counties and the waiting lists for individual homes may be long. Visits by family members to the homes are recommended prior to placement.

- Medicaid Eligibility. Operated by the local DSS. This service is available to anyone wishing to make an application. (See the section on Medicaid coverage for additional information.)

- Medicaid-Community Alternatives Program (CAP). Screening and case management operated differently in each county. These services are available to Medicaid and SNF/ICF eligible patients who can be adequately supported in the community (with appropriate services) and desire to remain in the community. Nurse-social worker teams are generally responsible for assessing the patient and the home situation and making a recommended plan of care. Medicaid funds can be used on health services to prevent or delay the institutionalization of Medicaid-eligible persons.

- Public Housing. Generally operated by the local housing authority. Services include rent subsidies and high-rise apartments and housing centers for the handicapped and elderly. Waiting lists for these housing services are long and the person must be fairly independent in order to qualify for these opportunities. Rates for housing are generally based on a sliding scale and ability to pay. Applications should be made to the housing authority.

- Meals on Wheels. Operated by a variety of agencies in various counties. Services typically include one meal delivered to the home on a daily basis (at least Monday to Friday). The meal is usually sponsored by public funds or private contributions. Costs run between $2.50 and $3.00 for each meal. Waiting lists are usually short, and the service also provides a daily check-in system for disabled homebound elders.

- Telephone Reassurance. Usually operated by the local Dept/ Div/Council on Aging. This service is a daily telephone check-in service run by volunteers. It primarily serves older adults with multiple health problems who are homebound and living alone.

- Loan Closet. Usually operated by the local Dept/Div/Council on Aging. This program keeps used medical equipment donated by other families and lends this equipment out to families/older people in need of assistance (see Equipment section for more information).

- Weatherization. Usually operated by the local Dept/Div/Council on Aging. This program is designed to help low-income elderly improve the insulation in their homes. Some agencies also provide emergency or routine assistance with fuel needs. Some programs require advance registration, and funds tend to be very limited. Generally, the work and the supplies are provided for a minimal fee or free of charge to qualified elders.

- RSVP. Operated as part of Federal Volunteer Agency, Retired Senior Volunteer Program (RSVP), uses the skills and abilities of community dwelling elders to help others. There are generally a wide variety of options for involvement. This program can be extremely beneficial to the older person experiencing role loss and the programs that reap the rewards of the services of the older persons. Some of the tasks can be done from the home and some require almost no physical stamina, others involve work with children in school classrooms, and so on.

- Transportation. Usually operated by the local Dept/Div/Council on Aging or the DSS. Van or bus transportation is sometimes available for physician appointments, shopping, attendance at nutritional and senior center programs, and other special events. There is generally some cost for the service, but some communities use local funding to provide the services for low-income persons. Arrangements must be made in advance to ensure the availability of transportation, and persons must be able to travel alone or have a helper with them.

Eligibility for each program varies with individual requirements. Further information about criteria for admission in any program can be obtained by contacting the sponsoring agency in the community.

Site Programs

There are a large number of programs offered to elderly individuals at centralized locations in the community. Programs demonstrate a wide array of options for assistance and support. Program quality and size varies greatly from one community to another. It pays to know the local resources before making referrals.

Programs include volunteer efforts, publicly funded services, nonprofit organizations, and privately owned for-profit programs. The availability of transportation to and from programs is a major factor in the accessibility and usefulness of these services to many impaired elders. Programs include:

- Support Groups. Activity centers where individuals with minimal to moderate impairments can gather for discussions, programs, games, crafts, planned outings, and congregate for meals. Hours vary, as does the presence of professional and volunteer staff to assist with programming. Participation is usually voluntary and free of charge.
- Nutrition Sites. Daily noon meals are provided in central locations. Donations are requested. Individuals need to be able to

get to and from the center and to feed themselves. The food is not typically tailored to special diets, but it does provide a majority of needed nutrients for at least one meal a day.

- Adult Day Care Centers. Daily supervision, programmed activities, and a noon meal are provided for minimally to moderately impaired elders. This service allows family members to work outside the home or offers some respite for full-time caregivers. Costs are in the $15 to $25/day range. The training of the staff may vary greatly, and sites should be visited if the program is being considered as part of a daily program for a patient. Admission criteria often include continence, transfer ability, nonwandering behavior, and nonaggressive behavior. Waiting lists tend to be rather long, and daily placement may not be available.

- Adult Day Health Centers. This program is a newly developed variation on the day care model. It is intended to provide services to more severely impaired individuals. Most states have developed some guidelines and regulations for these facilities. Availability will be limited for several years, until the programs get started.

- Outpatient Rehabilitation Services. Rehabilitation services are available through the hospital, in private practices, and in comprehensive outpatient rehabilitation facilities. Payment for services may be made through Medicare, Medicaid, private insurance, or private funds. Transportation to and from the facility and the limited coverage of insurance programs limit the usefulness of these programs for many older persons. These services cannot be used in conjunction with home-health services in most cases.

Eligibility for each program is generally determined by decisions of the organizations sponsoring the programs. Eligibility information can be obtained by contacting the agency in question.

Service Availability

Usually the best source for availability of services in your community is through your religious organization. Not only are these professionals trained to counsel you, but they have access to the many programs available and can help you decide which program might be best for your situation.

Most communities have some program to assist the mature adult whether it is a senior's support group, Meals on Wheels, health-related group, or other. Use Checklist 8 to locate which should be available to you.

■ MEDICARE PARTICIPATING PHYSICIAN

The Medicare participating physician has agreed to take assignment and file all Medicare claims for all services provided to the Medicare

---

CHECKLIST 8

Federal

Medicaid
Medicare
Social Security

State

Health and Rehabilitative Services

County

Programs for the aging
Health Departments
Local religious organizations

Housing

Adult Foster Homes - HRS
CARES - HRS
Adult Congregate Living Facilities - HRS

Medical

American Cancer Society
American Diabetes Association
American Heart Association
Arthritis Foundation
County Medical Association

Nutritional

American Dietetic Association
Meals on Wheels
Neighborly Senior Services

Services for the Hearing Impaired

Deaf Service Center
Vocational Rehabilitation Deaf Program - HRS

Services for the Sight Impaired

Division of Blind Services - HRS
National Society to Prevent Blindness

Services for the Physically Impaired

Decals and Stickers - County Tag Agency
Homemaker Services - HRS
The Disability Rights Education and Defense Fund (DREDF) (Write to this organization at DREDF, 1616 "P" Street, Northwest, Suite 100, Washington, DC 20036.)

Rehabilitative Services

Easter Seal Rehabilitation Services
Vocational Rehabilitation Services HRS

Transportation

Medicaid transportation
Wheelchair transport
American Red Cross
AARP—Local Chapters

patient. This usually means a lower cost to the patient over the nonassignment provider. The patient is responsible for the $75 annual deductible and 20 percent of the approved charges as co-payment for all services except laboratory procedures. All providers of laboratory services must accept Medicare assignment and have agreed to reduce their charges to the amount paid by Medicare with no co-payment from the patient for this service. Most Medigap Supplemental Coverage will pick up the 20 percent of approved charge co-payment (rarely the $75 deductible). Certain services are not covered by Medicare (influenza injections, etc.) and will be the patient's responsibility.

■ MEDICARE NONPARTICIPATING PHYSICIAN

This physician may elect to accept assignment on a case-by-case basis except for laboratory services that are always on assignment from all providers and at no cost to the patient. When assignment is not accepted, the patient will be responsible for the billed amount, but if more than the Medicare approved amount will cost the patient the difference *plus the 20 percent co-payment*. Medigap coverage will not usually cover this difference. For example, the provider might bill $200 with Medicare approving $180 of the amount. Under assignment, the patient is responsible for 20 percent of $180 or $36 which Medigap coverage should pay. Without assignment, the patient would be responsible for $200 less $180 or $20 plus the $36 co-payment or $56 with Medigap picking up only $36. When the billed charge is more than the approved charge and assignment is not taken then the patient can be responsible for the difference plus co-payment (except lab charges).

■ HEALTH MAINTENANCE ORGANIZATION (HMO)

The HMO concept is being offered by more companies and as an optional plan with traditional insurance companies. Deciding to choose this provider of medical care requires that we understand its makeup.

While the HMO's choice of care might best preserve the patient's assets in case of a serious illness, in doing so it also offers the patient the least control over his or her medical care. Take a long look at HMOs before you get involved.

The HMO receives its income from the employer and/or the government (Medicare) plus in some cases a co-payment from the patient. To attract patients, the HMO usually offers additional services that might include prescription drugs (sometimes with co-payment), some dental, hearing aids, and eyeglasses.

From the fixed income received each month, the HMO must pay for all of the patient's services both as an outpatient and/or as an in-hospital patient. HMOs experienced rapid growth over the past 10 years with national enrollment in 1988 of approximately 30 million people. Of those, about 1.7 million were Medicare beneficiaries. Recent enrollment has slowed down as many HMOs are experiencing financial difficulties with some becoming insolvent. When the HMO loses money, it is forced to cut back on services and/or increase its co-payment while attempting to increase its income by charging more for its services to the employees and/or government (Medicare) when possible. The patient will then experience a cut-back in the services provided. The patient might see other professionals (RN, physician's assistant) more and the physician less. The use of specialists would be discouraged, surgery postponed, and marginal hospital admissions delayed. Many states are requiring increased financial reserves for HMOs and are establishing guidelines for standard of care. The Omnibus Reconciliation Act of 1987 has a provision requiring Health Care Financing Administration to draft regulations that force HMOs to cover Medicare beneficiaries for up to six months after they withdraw or have their contacts terminated by Medicare. The Medicare patient should carefully consider whether to cancel his or her Medigap coverage upon joining the HMO. Should you later decide to drop out of the HMO and re-enter Medicare and obtain new Medigap coverage, a pre-existing condition might require a waiting period for it to be covered.

Carefully consider this provider of health care that offers elimination of deductibles and in some cases a small co-payment. The trade-off is that you will have less control of your health care. You will see only the HMO physician and be admitted only to the HMO hospital. In most cases, your HMO physician will control the services you receive.

The HMO offers the potential for the lowest cost but also the *least* control over your medical care.

■ INDIVIDUAL PRACTICE ASSOCIATION (IPA)

The IPA was developed by office-based physicians to meet the competitive threat of the conventional HMOs that were receiving federal government support.

The IPA is a prepaid health plan or HMO that typically reimburses member providers (physicians and hospitals) reduced fees for service basis. The conventional HMO usually has staff physicians on their panel and limited clinic-type facilities. The patient using an IPA would have a greater choice of physicians and possibly a more convenient office to visit. The IPA in principle can be started with less capital by utilizing the existing IPA member facilities. The patient might find this type of HMO more attractive as it usually offers greater selection of physicians and offices. Most employer plans will offer this option of coverage. The patient's cost is usually less with no deductible, but often has a co-payment that can vary with the plan. Many of the IPA plans have experienced financial difficulties in recent years. One making this choice should be sure that the plan is financially sound. This choice again might offer less cost to the patient but also will restrict the patient's choice of providers of quality medical care.

■ PREFERRED PROVIDER ORGANIZATION (PPO)

Most insurance companies are now offering the option of a PPO for medical care.

This type of organization is becoming a means to provide medical care under somewhat controlled circumstances. The term *pre-certification* will become a popular term in delivering health care services. The PPO is usually made up of a group of providers that are willing to accept reduced fees for services in return for additional patients. In choosing this option, the patient usually will find the deductible waived and co-payment reduced from 20 to 10 percent. This should reduce the patient's out-of-pocket expense. The trade-off is that the choice of a provider of services must be from the panel of PPO providers. In addition, nonemergency admissions to the hospital must be precertified with usually a second opinion for surgery. The PPO will be involved in the patient's care. The use of a specialist must be pre-approved and when possible limited to a physician on the PPO panel. The use of a nonapproved physician or hospital can result in a higher deductible and co-payment or possibly no payment at all. This encourages the patient to use PPO providers.

This program offers a lower out-of-pocket cost when using the PPO providers only but the trade-off is less control over your health care. If your personal physician or choice of a hospital is not on the panel, it might cause you to have second thoughts before making this choice.

■ HOME EQUITY CONVERSION

Many adults upon retirement prefer staying in their initial homes yet find a great need for additional cash. If this is your situation, you might consider the "Home Equity Conversion" commonly called reverse mortgage. Most areas of the country should have at least one of these plans available by 1990. The plan will offer to pay a fixed amount each month for a set period at which time the house would be sold and the loan repaid. This is a new idea which seems to be catching on, but the plan can vary as to terms and conditions and should receive careful review before signing a contract. The plan can offer a fixed amount each month for 5 to 10 years and might offer the lender an interest in any property appreciation. With the participation in appreciation, the retiree might be permitted to stay in the home for a longer period.

U.S. Department of Housing and Urban Development (HUD) is planning to enter the picture with insurance being proposed for three types of loans, including:

- Split Term—A lender makes payment for a specific term agreed upon when the loan is originated. The borrower may stay in the house after the term expires but the lender will not make any additional payments and interest continues to accrue on the amount paid out.
- Line of Credit—Rather than getting a check each month, a homeowner can draw funds as special needs arise.
- Tenual—A borrower receives checks as long as he or she is in the house. Should a lender's payments to the homeowner plus accumulated interest exceed the property value, the consumer's liability is limited to the value of the house. The difference would be covered by the FHA insurance fund.

Under the HUD experiment, the maximum loan amounts will be the same as in current FHA single-family home mortgage programs from $67,500 to $101,250.

The HUD insurance program is just part of the stepped up reverse mortgage activity. Plan to stay current with HUD's proposed plans for this area. The private sector is also moving rapidly to set up similar plans. All of this is good news for house rich, cash poor older Americans who have been waiting for reverse mortgages to become available. But it will not be a panacea. Mature adults are advised to talk things over with a third party before entering into a reverse mortgage situation. Higher interest for this type financing and placing a loan on our home should receive serious consideration before entering this type of contract.

■ HOME EQUITY (SALE)

Should the mature adult decide to sell the home in order to put the finishing touches on financing the retirement plan, consideration must be given to the tax liability on any profit. Again, be sure to discuss this thoroughly with your financial advisor before you decide to sell. The profit is taxable income under the present law and there is no automatic exclusion of a portion of any capital gain.

When certain conditions are met, any tax on the gain is deferred as long as you purchase a replacement dwelling that costs at least as much as your present residence sold for. You must purchase the new home within 24 months after the old one is sold. Should your new home cost less than the adjusted selling price of your old home, you must pay the tax on the profit from the sale on the portion of the sale price that exceeds the cost of the new home or whichever is less.

Adjusting the sales price of the old home to reflect finance points, any cost to fix up, real estate commissions, and legal fees will assist in reducing any tax obligation.

You are exposed to this tax anytime you purchase a primary residence whose price exceeds the adjusted sale price of your old home.

The over-55 tax break offers the mature adult the chance to sell the house and avoid tax on the first $125,000 of profits, *but only once in a lifetime.*

You must qualify for this tax break by living in your principal residence for at least three of the last five years before the sale.

Congress passed a tax bill in 1988 that provides for two minor changes to this law. First, a couple will not be denied the benefits of the deferral because one spouse dies after the old home has been sold, but before the new home is purchased.

The second change covers that person who is 55 or older who becomes mentally or physically incapable of self-care during the five-year period preceding the house sale. This person will be deemed to have met the residency requirements if up to four of the five years are spent in a nursing home.

Before you sell your home, discuss the pros and cons of selling and the tax effects on your estate with your financial advisor.

■ SUPPLEMENTING YOUR INCOME

Every mature adult needs to ask, Do I plan to supplement my income with part-time work? Before working part-time, review the section on Social Security and become aware of the effect that part-time earnings will have on your Social Security. A growing number of businesses are finding that part-time mature adults make excellent and dependable employees. The business office, fast food restaurants, grocery stores, department stores, religious institutions, senior citizens centers, and so on offer excellent opportunities for part-time employment.

■ NURSING HOMES

Booklets are available to provide you with information on nursing homes and nursing home insurance from the following sources:

1. Health Insurance Association of America has a free booklet entitled "The Consumer's Guide to Long-Term Care Insurance." This guide has a checklist to compare costs and provisions of policies while assisting you in making decisions as to the best policy. Write—HIAA, P.O. Box 41455, Washington, DC 20018.

2. The American Association of Homes for the Aging, 1129 20th Street, SW, Suite 400, Washington, DC 20036, represents about 3500 nonprofit retirement communities and nursing homes. It offers several free pamphlets and through state affiliates, offers some guidance on local options. "The Continuing Care Retirement Community: A Guidebook for the Consumers," costs $2.00 prepaid. The association is also considering a group long-term care policy to be offered through its member communities.

■ THE WILL IS FOR ALL PEOPLE

As you establish retirement goals, it is necessary that you periodically update your will. It has been estimated that up to 60 percent of all adults do not have a will. This can be one of the most important decisions a mature adult or any adult for that matter can make. Rather than have the court decide how to divide your estate at tremendous costs, it is important to have a properly drawn will in order to carry out your instructions upon your death.

The cost for a simple will should be reasonable and should range from $100 to $200. Other estate planning tools such as joint ownership and living trusts could increase the cost somewhat, but the results are still most cost-effective.

Your will should be reviewed periodically as your estate changes or should you move to another state. Your attorney can best advise you and prepare this vital document.

■ MAKE CHECKLISTS

Financial advisors strongly recommend a detailed list of everything a survivor needs to know upon death of the person. Without this list, your loved ones will spend needless time in searching for the information.

- Insurance. List your agents including the phone number for each policy. List policies by name, address, type of coverage including business coverage.
- Will and Important Papers. List the location of your will (a copy sent to your executor, accountant, etc. is advisable). Also list the following locations of birth certificates, marriage certificates, military discharge, business agreements, mortgages, deeds, titles for automobiles, all bank accounts, recent tax returns.
- Advisors. List your advisors by name and phone number including the following key individuals: Religious leader, accountant, insurance agent, attorney, financial planner, bank officer, employer, executor, and/or any other important player in your life.
- Assets. Inventory all of your assets and their location on this key list. If titles are involved, write down their location. For all cash, and stocks and bonds, list the financial institutions, type of account and account number, and location of any savings books. Also list any safe deposit boxes, location of the keys, person with access to these, and an inventory of the contents.
- Debts. List all credit cards, the issuers and phone numbers. Make a list of your home mortgage, auto loans, and any personal loans. List anyone else that you owe money to including monthly living expenses.

As you review your will from time to time, also review this list and update as needed. Any special instructions could be left with this list so be certain that your spouse or family member is familiar with it and knows its location.

■ WHEN A SPOUSE DIES

When your partner dies, there are many financial details to be taken care of. Some of these arrangements are immediate and others can be put off for several months until a more appropriate time. Checklist 9 will give you guidelines to follow when this situation happens to you.

■ HELP IS AVAILABLE

In addition to the federal programs available for mature adults through Social Security and Medicare, you need to become acquainted with many other sources of assistance.

As you approach 50, a good source of information on aging is available by joining the AARP and paying an annual membership of only $5.00. The membership offers the following:

- MODERN MATURITY magazine
- 11 issues of the AARP News Bulletin
- Free retirement planning information
- Eligibility for group health insurance
- Legislative representation in Washington
- Savings on pharmacy products
- Hotel, motel, car rental, and air travel discounts
- Investment program
- Auto and homeowner insurance opportunities
- Federal Credit Union
- Volunteer opportunities
- Eligibility for local chapter membership

You can write for membership in the AARP to P.O. Box 199, Long Beach, CA 90801-0199.

Other publications that may assist you in retirement planning include: *Money* magazine and *Consumer Reports*.

Other Resources

There are numerous resources available free of charge to the public on issues concerning the older adult. We have listed just a few of the agencies that you can write to ask for free brochures on retirement, pension plans, legal rights, and more.

CHECKLIST 9

WHEN A SPOUSE DIES

_____ Find instructions for the funeral and burial by the deceased person. Were organs donated to science? Did the deceased want to be cremated? If so, follow through with these plans as indicated in the written will or separate letter.

_____ Order a dozen certified copies of the death certificate from the county clerk's office or from the funeral director. You will use these certified copies to claim death benefits and Social Security, and to retitle joint assets and properties.

_____ File the will in probate court after your attorney has had an opportunity to review it.

_____ Apply for death benefits. Call your insurance agent, your spouse's employer, and your local Social Security office. You will need to take with you the following documents: your marriage certificate and both of your birth certificates.

_____ As money begins to come in from insurance policies and other benefits, deposit this income in short-term bank certificates of deposit. This is not the time to think about investments and the money will earn some interest while locked-in a guaranteed fund.

_____ Change all beneficiary designations in your will and on all insurance policies, investments, retirement plans, and other that named your spouse as beneficiary. Also let the appropriate people know you want the names changed on any joint accounts.

_____ Satisfy debts and notify creditors. Be sure to verify any debt notices you receive as you will be vulnerable to pranks during this time.

_____ Make certain all estate taxes are paid. You must file federal estate taxes within nine months of the death if the estate is larger than $600,000. You must also pay the estate's income taxes due April 15th for every year the estate is open.

You must be aware of the many sources of potential financial assistance that are available for burial expenses. Check into the following sources _before_ death of spouse to see if you qualify:

_____ U.S. Social Security/Canada Pension Benefit

_____ Veteran's Administration

_____ Department of Veteran Affairs (Canada)

_____ Union or Employer Pension Funds

_____ Insurance

_____ Fraternal Orders or Professional Groups

_____ Workman's Compensation

- Pension Rights Center
  1346 Connecticut Avenue, NW
  Washington, DC 20036

- Age Discrimination Project
  American Association of Retired Persons
  1909 K Street, NW
  Washington, DC 20049

- Association of Employment Services for the Elderly
  National Council on the Aging
  1828 L Street
  Washington, DC 20036

- Administration on Aging
  Publication Department
  Room 4146
  330 Independence Avenue, SW
  Washington, DC 20201

- American Association of Retired Persons
  P.O. Box 2240
  Long Beach, CA 90801

Nursing Home Information

- How to Select a Nursing Home
  Superintendent of Documents
  U.S. Government Printing Office
  Washington, DC 20402

- American Nursing Home Association
  American Health Care Association
  1025 Connecticut Avenue, NW
  Washington, DC 20036

For home care opportunities in your area, obtain from:

- National Home Care Council
  67 Irving Place
  New York, NY 10003

- National Health Information Clearinghouse
  P.O. Box 1133
  Washington, DC 20013

For information on psychological problems, a list of community mental health centers in your area is available from:

- National Institute of Mental Health
  5600 Fishers Lane
  Room 214-21
  Rockville, MD 20857

Pamphlets available from the local Social Security office include:

1. An Introduction to Social Security
2. Part of Your Benefits May Be Taxable
3. Retirement
4. Your Social Security Earnings Record
5. Financial Planning and Social Security
6. Estimating Your Social Security Check
7. When and How to Contact Social Security
8. Social Security "How It Works for You"
9. How We Decide If You Are Still Disabled
10. Retiring? Remember Social Security
11. History of Social Security
12. Form W-2 Annual Wage Report Checklist
13. If You Get Benefits from Social Security
14. Your Social Security Checks While You Are Outside of the United States
15. Medicare for Federal Employees
16. How Your Social Security Check Is Affected by Workers' Compensation and Public Disability Payments
17. Medicare and Medicaid
18. Medicare and Employer Health Plans
19. Your Right to Appeal Your Medical Insurance Payment
20. Hospice Benefits Under Medicare
21. Medicare and Prepayment Plans
22. Thinking of Having Surgery
23. Filing for Disability Benefits
24. Filing for Social Security or Supplement Security Income Disability Benefits
25. Disability

New publications are being printed frequently. Ask for new publications when you call your Social Security office.

CHECKLIST 10

PERSONAL ASSISTANCE

Key people and organizations who can help you in your mature years should be listed on this form. Keep the phone numbers updated on a yearly basis.

	Name	*Phone*
Accountant	_____	_____
Lawyer	_____	_____
Financial planner	_____	_____
Banker	_____	_____
Religious counselor	_____	_____
Physician	_____	_____
Dentist	_____	_____
Other	_____	_____

Insurance company	*Agent*	*Phone*
_____	_____	_____
_____	_____	_____
_____	_____	_____
_____	_____	_____

Public assistance agency	*Person*	*Phone*
_____	_____	_____
_____	_____	_____
_____	_____	_____
_____	_____	_____

Other service	*Person*	*Phone*
_____	_____	_____
_____	_____	_____
_____	_____	_____
_____	_____	_____

CHECKLIST 11

PERSONAL NET WORTH FORM

Retain this statement and compare each year with the previous year to determine your financial progress. Alter your plan as needed to fulfill the required assets to meet your goal. This form is for you to fill out using your figures.

	Current Year *Amount*	_____ *Year* *Amount*
Assets—What You Own		
1. Retirement Plan incl. IRA	_____	_____
2. Total Bank Funds (cash)	_____	_____
3. Other income investments (bonds, CDs, etc.)	_____	_____
4. Common Stocks including Mutual Funds	_____	_____
5. Real Estate Investment (market value) equity	_____	_____
6. Other Investments—Business interest, collectibles, other	_____	_____
7. Net Value of Business	_____	_____
8. Market Value of Home	_____	_____
9. Life Insurance Cash Value	_____	_____
10. Personal Property, i.e., furniture, jewelry, etc.	_____	_____
11. Automobile(s)	_____	_____
12. Miscellaneous (money owed to you, security deposits, etc.)	_____	_____
13. Total Assets—What you own	_____	_____
Add items (1) thru (12)	_____	_____
Liabilities—What You Owe		
14. Balance on Mortgage(s)	_____	_____
15. Taxes Due	_____	_____
16. Auto Loans	_____	_____
17. Other Loans	_____	_____

CHECKLIST 11 (*Continued*)

	Current Year Amount	_____ Year Amount
18. Monthly Bills (Credit Cards) & other short term obligations	_____	_____
19. Total Liabilities Total (14) thru (18)	_____	_____
20. Net Worth (13) less (19)	_____	_____

CHECKLIST 12

PERSONAL EXPENSE FORM

The following Expense Form is for you to fill out using your specific figures.

Expenses	Current Year	Changes- Retirement
1. Housing mortgage, taxes, utilities, electricity, water, gas & oil	_____	_____
2. Food incl. entertaining at home	_____	_____
3. Transportation, payments, repairs, food & other	_____	_____
4. Clothing & linens	_____	_____
5. Insurance—Property, auto, health, life	_____	_____
6. Medical & Dental—out of pocket	_____	_____
7. Contributions & gifts	_____	_____
8. Repayment of loans—credit cards, etc.	_____	_____
9. Recreation—entertainment, vacations, sports events, hobbies, etc.	_____	_____
10. Miscellaneous expenses	_____	_____
11. Savings & retirement IRAs, company plan, investments, other	_____	_____
12. Taxes (Local, State, Federal)	_____	_____
13. Total Expenses	_____	_____
14. Total Reduction for Retirement	_____	_____
15. Projected Expenses for Retirement—Line 13 Less 14	_____	_____

CHAPTER 10

A Healthy
Attitude

During the mature years, we must make decisions that focus on how we will respond to the guaranteed life changes that will take place. This stage in life may prompt us to face some limitations as we may face unexpected illnesses, death of a spouse or loved one, or declining mobility. These life changes during our older years can cause sorrow and depression. But these guaranteed life changes don't have to dominate our thoughts day-in and day-out. In fact, this stage in life can allow us to have more opportunity than ever before to explore our potential as we experience more free time, mobility to live anywhere we choose, and less responsibility to care for dependents.

In order to understand the total life cycle, we must look at aging as an ongoing process that takes place throughout our entire life. People do not merely wake up at a certain age and determine that they are now "old." In fact, we all know those amazing people who are active and vibrant in their eighties and nineties, and wonder what their secret is! We also know too well those people who seem to be very "old" in their forties and fifties, having lost that enthusiasm for living.

Age is like that. People really don't grow old by merely living a certain number of years. Old age is of the mind. People grow old when they quit taking risks in their lives; when they lose their zest for waking each morning; when they ignore their dreams and allow their lives to become mundane and lackluster.

Unlike the young adult who is constantly exploring his potential or the middle adult who is in the process of re-examining his life, the older adult usually lives with the result of the many choices made throughout his lifetime. For some mature adults, those dreams that began years ago are now being seen as a reality as they capture their creativity in hobbies, second careers, travel, volunteering, and other meaningful uses of free time. Many mature adults are realizing new dreams as they find hidden talents and meet new friends. Yet for other mature adults, the adage "nothing ventured, nothing gained" becomes a reality as their retirement years are spent in mundane activities because of lack of personal planning and lack of vision.

Often mature adults put aside those dreams that began in their younger years, and a new dream is formed. Gifted artist Grandma Moses did not even begin her career until age 76 and even painted 25 works the year after her 100th birthday! While she may have been considered "old" by society's standards, she was actually just being born by following her new dream and living each day with expectation as she expressed herself through a creative medium.

Imagine waking up each morning expecting something new and positive to happen in your life! Yes, it is an attitude that must be chosen by you, but it can also govern your overall well-being allowing for continued growth in the mature years. Depression can also govern one's well-being and is a reality for many mature adults as they begin to feel quite limited by the number of years left in their life calendar. This depression and worry can be a contributing factor to many types of stress-related diseases. Some older adults begin to dwell on these limitations and worries such as declining mobility, fixed income, or health problems. Yet, for many mature adults who are living their retirement years to the fullest, these limitations are accepted and affirmed as part of the changing lifestyle. These adults who live their mature years positively and to the fullest are the ones who dwell not on their limitations, but on their capabilities, talents, wisdom, and especially the knowledge gained through the many years of life.

Instead of focusing only on the limitations that may accompany the life changes of the mature years, let us look at how we can affirm these changes and use these years to capture a sense of discovery of self and those around us.

■ ATTITUDE CHECK

Sofie is a seventy-year-old widow living alone in a small town in the south. She has had her share of misfortune through the years. Her only son was killed in Vietnam, and her husband died ten years ago after a lengthy illness which virtually absorbed all of Sofie's savings. She now lives alone with her two cats on a fixed income—Social Security and a small pension from her husband's career with the railroad. But Sofie doesn't feel alone or sorry for herself in any way. In fact, this woman recently won the Volunteer of the Year award for the public school system in her town. She prides herself in going to the small elementary school near her home each day at 8:00 A.M. and running the school clinic. As a retired home health nurse, Sofie's talents and abilities were not put aside in the mature years. She is still giving of herself and receiving even more in knowing that she is needed by the children she cares for.

Then there is Bill—Bill is a retired executive from a large paper manufacturing plant in the midwest. Having never married, Bill gave his life to his company and worked many hours each day to move up the corporate structure. Upon retirement at age 66, Bill was a senior vice president—the highest office anyone could have next to chairman of the board. But Bill had some difficulties. Throughout his young adult and middle years, he had neglected to do anything else but work. He had no hobbies, no spouse, no friends, and no direction when he left his company. Bill now sits day-in and day-out in his worn recliner watching game shows on television and dwelling on the "good old days" when he had a purpose in life.

■ WHAT IS YOUR ATTITUDE?

How about you? How is your attitude toward the mature years? toward retirement? Did you know that what you say and how you act has a great influence on your life and on those around you? Your thoughts, feelings, and behavior mirror your soul. If you are full of depressing thoughts, doubts, and suspicions, then your life becomes negative. But if you are enthusiastic, hopeful, and positive, your mature years can be filled with meaning and have a vibrant impression on those around you.

What you think each day, how you act and react to situations, and what you say to those around you—all govern your overall perspective on life. Most people usually move from crises to crises in all stages in their lives; yes, including the young adult and middle years. Yet, it is how you look at these crises that determine their outcome. To one person, an illness may become a tremendous burden with no hope for recovery. To another person with a positive outlook on life, the same illness could be viewed as time for personal reflection as time is spent on reading, letter writing, or talking with friends. While death becomes a reality for many mature adults, it is a reality for all humankind and should be accepted as such instead of waiting for it to occur. Yet you would be surprised at how many perfectly healthy mature adults sit at home wanting sympathy from family and friends as they wait in fear for "their time to come."

Your expectations can determine the path your life as a mature adult will take. As you become more knowledgeable about the realities of aging as a lifetime process, you can learn to accept the changing stages in your life as part of a natural plan. Once you accept these changing stages, it is time to move on with great expectation and discover what each day can unfold for you.

Additional Reading

Suggestions for additional reading are included. A complete list of references is available on request to the authors through the publisher.

Gruetzner, Howard. 1988. *Alzheimer's: A Caregiver's Guide and Sourcebook.* New York: Wiley.

Hurst, J.W. 1988. *Medicine for the Practicing Physician.* (Stoneham, MA: Butterworth).

McIlwain, H.H., Bruce, D.F., Silverfield, J.C., Burnette, M.C. 1988. *Osteoporosis: Prevention, Management, Treatment.* (New York: Wiley).

National Cholesterol Education Program. 1988. *Report of the Expert Panel on Detection, Evaluation and Treatment of High Blood Cholesterol in Adults.* (Washington, D.C.: U.S. Department of Health and Human Services, Public Health Service, National Institutes of Health).

National High Blood Pressure Education Program. 1988. *The 1988 Report of the Joint National Committee on Detection, Evaluation, and Treatment of High Blood Pressure.* (Washington, D.C.: U.S. Department of Health and Human Services, Public Health Services, National Institutes of Health).

Neidrick, Darla J. 1988. *Caring for Your Own: Nursing the Ill at Home.* New York: Wiley.

Rossman, I. 1986. The Anatomy of Aging. In I. Rossman, *Clinical Geriatrics.* (Philadelphia: Lippincott). p. 3–20.

Russell, Charles H., Ph.D. in association with Anthony P. Russell, Ph.D. and Inger Megaad, RN: *Good News About Aging,* New York: John Wiley & Sons, 1989.

U.S. Department of Health and Human Services, Public Health Service, National Institutes of Health. 1986. *Clinical Opportunities for Smoking Intervention.* (Washington, D.C.: U.S. Government Printing Office).

Index